Special Deliveries

A Surgeon's Story of Birth, Death, and Learning to See

Kevin Kington, M.D.

and

Jas Scarff

Olentangy River Press

First printing

ISBN-13: 978-1727819403

ISBN-10: 1727819403

Printed in the United States of America

I dedicate this book to Nancy because without

her love and support, it would have been

impossible to pursue my dreams. ~ Kevin

For Toni Johnson.

Big sister; best friend. ~ Jas

Contents

Prologue

lood. I've been an obstetrician-gynecologist for thirty years and birth is a bloody process. C-sections are even worse. Except, perhaps, for trauma surgery, there is no field of medicine where you see so much of it. There's a saying among ob-gyn docs that it's really not heavy bleeding until you can hear it. Early on this morning, I heard it.

I got to the hospital by 7:00 for our morning conference. I'm the supervisor of ob-gyn residents at a Midwest suburban hospital, and the morning conference lets the residents talk about what happened the night before, what's happening on the floor right now, and any difficult cases that need special attention. We gathered, as usual, around an empty nurses' station with our coffee, talking over the patient summaries on the big screen. One resident, Cynthia West, was concerned about a young patient in her first pregnancy. Florence had been in labor, delivered the baby, and everything was fine. Then she started to bleed. Heavily.

The second-year resident on duty the night before, Tom Lear, had assisted the attending physician with the delivery and they found a mass in the uterus that they thought was a benign tumor called a fibroid. So they gave Florence medication to make the uterus clamp down to stop the bleeding. It slowed, but it didn't stop, and she was so low on blood that she went into shock. They transfused her and sent her to the ICU.

Cynthia told us what she heard from Tom when she came on duty. That's when the bells started ringing in my head. I had heard this same story three or four times in my career. Right after a delivery the patient tries to pass a fibroid and has heavy bleeding. But every time I'd heard that story it turned out to be wrong. The fibroid turned out to be something else entirely — a uterine inversion. Bad news. The uterus turns inside out as the placenta is delivered and the bleeding begins. All the vessels of the uterus are exposed and you've got massive hemorrhaging.

What you need to do and do quickly is to go in and turn the uterus right side out. That's hard to do. So is convincing doctors that they're wrong.

"That patient has an inverted uterus," I said.

"No, no, Tom's sure it's a prolapsing fibroid. The patient's in the ICU now and she's stable." Cynthia's phone rang. It was the ICU.

By the time we got down there the new mother was near death. Florence had lost about two-thirds of her blood and was close to entering a dangerous state called DIC. The medical term is Disseminated Intravascular Coagulation, but I sometimes think of it as Death Is Coming. You can bleed so heavily that the stuff that makes your blood clot is gone. And you are, too. You bleed out.

Cynthia's a good doctor and when she had scrubbed and began working with the patient it became clear to her that she was dealing with something she had never seen — an inverted uterus. This patient teetered on a knife edge: still bleeding, facing possible DIC, and caught between the conflicting demands this condition presents. The doctor must administer short-term drugs that relax the uterus so that it can be manipulated and turned right side out. But relaxation increases bleeding, so the uterus must be repositioned quickly and held firmly to minimize that bleeding until the relaxant wears off. The balance is tricky and timing is crucial.

The dance of a surgical procedure is a subtle one. There's not much talk and movements quickly revert to rote. An empty hand is extended and the hand holding an instrument is withdrawn. Vital signs are read without request. Experience is forged into its most basic shape; what once was thought is now habit.

We had a good team: Cynthia, the attending physician, me, a couple of nurses, and the assistants running blood and supplies into the OR. It wasn't easy. The uterus refused to reposition correctly, and Cynthia struggled. I could have stepped in if it was necessary, but learning how to do this would allow her to save another patient someday. I learned under the gun. Cynthia was learning under the gun. That's medicine.

She got it done with a combination of persistence and exasperation — and a lot of transfusions. Nature furnishes a pregnant woman with more blood than the rest of us — about 6 liters instead of 5 — and we had replaced far more than that, along with a lot of the stuff that makes the blood clot. Finally, the patient stabilized and we went, with spattered scrubs, back to rounds. It was a long morning.

Cynthia will never hear the diagnosis of a prolapsing fibroid in the same way. She gained an indelible lesson from this case, and over the years I gained many lessons by having opportunities to watch docs like her. Unlike someone in private practice, I've had the luxury as a supervisor to learn from the experiences of all the doctors I worked with and to see what hundreds of doctors saw. From them I've learned that seeing what is happening in front of you is harder than you think. We tend to default to what we've experienced before. In medicine, that can be useful common sense. A famous medical proverb, after all, warns us about getting too fancy with a diagnosis: "If you hear hoof beats, don't look for zebras." Good advice. But zebras are out there, and a patient's life might depend on recognizing one. Tom Lear had seen fibroids before — they're fairly common — so he saw a horse when he examined Florence when he should have been considering zebras. And he convinced Cynthia.

Experience is a useful collection of events, a library of memories that we can dip into for guidance. But experience without perspective restricts us to those specific memories without any chance for greater insight. Doctors need to know when to look past what they've seen before, past those things that they're projecting onto the present, to see what's there right now. In a curious way, the more you see and experience, the more you question what you're seeing. Rote procedure can get you out of a crisis. Previous cases can give you guidance and confidence. But at that point the most experienced physicians take a critical look and, if necessary, ignore their experience to see what's happening right there. A medical education is a collision between the comfortable certainties of the things that you think you know and the difficult necessities of what real life is trying to tell you.

I'm sure collisions occur in any education, but the difference in medicine is that the stakes are so high. I was terrified for much of my early residency and for good reason. The lives of strangers were in my hands. The journey from intimidated medical student to terrified intern to competent physician is a long one. It can be funny, frightening, and occasionally very moving. That's the story I want to tell here. For me, that journey began in an unconventional way a long time ago. The day was Monday, June 5, 1978.

☙

Apart from changing some names, places, and dates, this story is true as much as the limits of memory will allow.

Chapter 1

Coming Home

In Which Nancy and I Begin to Rewrite Our Script

In the summer of 1978 I had been married for five years. We got started early. I graduated from college a week before the wedding and my wife, Nancy, the day before. After five years, we had two kids, a mortgage, Nancy was pregnant with our third, and I hated my job.

I was working as an actuary for a very large insurance company, crunching the numbers that would tell us the odds of what might happen to which of our policyholders. I liked math and I liked actuarial work. The job had no stress but that was because it had no challenge. I was studying for professional exams, taking them, getting promotions, getting raises, and everything was going just great. I was on the fast track for having a corner office, lots of employees, and wanting to blow my brains out.

One of the exams I took was heavily medical — about medical underwriting — so there was a lot in it on how the heart works, on blood pressure, diabetes, and all sorts of diseases. I found it fascinating. As I was casting around for ways to change my life and make it more interesting I kept thinking about that medical exam.

Then, on June 5th, Nancy and I went to the movie *Coming Home* with Jon Voigt and Jane Fonda. In the movie, Voigt is a disabled Vietnam veteran in a wheelchair and he goes into a VA hospital. He's being cared for by various people and I thought, "Wouldn't it be great to make that much difference in somebody's life? Doctors really do make a difference. I think that's what I want to do."

At twenty-seven years old that was the first time I ever thought about being a doctor. I had absolutely no pre-med science in school. I graduated with a B.S. in mathematics and the only science I took was psychology. I hadn't taken biology, zoology, chemistry, physics — any of it. So I said all this to my wife at dinner after the movie and Nancy made the fatal mistake of saying, "You know, you could do whatever you set your mind to do." Boy, did she come to regret that statement.

The next morning we were down in the pre-med counseling office of the state university. What they had to say was far from encouraging. The counselor told me that med school doesn't like older students and that only great students would even be considered. She recommended that if I applied at all I should apply to a medical school in another part of the state that had a reputation for accepting "non-standard" students. I ignored her and studied for the MCATs and two years later, with great satisfaction, I took my scores and the acceptance letter from her med school around to show her.

That's a good memory but an even better memory of this whole crazy time is of my boss, Steve, at the insurance company. I went in to tell him what I was doing and assumed that I would be fired. But Steve said, "Well, how long is it going to take you to do all these science courses?" I told him that it would be about eighteen months, so he asked me why I couldn't work for them half-time while I was going to school and then I could get half my pay. That was crucial. It really made the dream practical. That wasn't the last time my boss would help me out on this new journey.

This was a period of great excitement but probably not of great prudence. Nancy and I had decided when we married that we wanted five kids and she made it clear that she still wanted that. I told her that I did, too, and that I would make her a promise. We would have the five kids, I would never flunk a course, and I would never make honors. That was our deal. There was always going to be family time along with the studies. As I look back at us standing on that frightening threshold I realize that each of us was more concerned than we let the other know. Let Nancy tell it.

When we first put our house on the market, that's when it became very real for me. We were going to sell the house and use whatever money we got out of it to get started with medical school. We would rent in the meantime, because we didn't know how it would go financially. I was more sad than I was scared. We loved that house. We were a good team though. That was the most important thing to me. I was twenty-six and Kevin was twenty-seven. We had done quite well at the insurance company, and we thought we could do this. I had a lot of confidence. I felt that we could make anything work. I've thought later that the amount of faith that I had in Kevin might have felt like a burden to him.

Actually the biggest burden for me was feeling so selfish. I was putting our young family's happiness on the line to satisfy my own needs and that didn't feel comfortable. But staying in my rut at the insurance company wasn't going to be healthy for me. I've always liked numbers, but I like people a lot more and I wasn't getting much personal contact at the insurance company.

Nancy said,

Kevin is a classic people person, so I wasn't surprised that the insurance company wasn't a good fit. I just didn't know that he was so unhappy. He kept that pretty much inside until after we saw the movie.

After the two of us talked it over, it was time to tell our families and that wasn't easy. Nancy's dad was scared. Henry was not a reticent man, but when we told him about our plans he clammed up for days. Our parents had all lived through the Great

Depression and knew how vulnerable a family could be to money problems. They could see the risks because they had lived them.

My dad said, "Kevin, you know those people in medical school are the cream of the crop."

This was from the guy who had been my biggest cheerleader growing up. He had annoyed countless parents at baseball and football games by bragging about me. "Kevin's got all the tools" was his mantra. When I heard the "cream of the crop" remark I didn't know whether to laugh or cry. Our families accepted the idea eventually, though until I made it through medical school a lot of doubts were expressed about my judgment. I shared them.

So I went back to school as a very unusual student. My first day in chemistry class I walked in wearing a powder-blue seventies suit and a tie, and I carried a Samsonite attaché case with all my actuarial work in it. The first student I saw, my eventual lab partner, said to me, "Do you have a copy of the syllabus? Is this course going to be graded on the curve?" I told him that I couldn't help him with either of those things, so he began asking me about electron shells. I confessed that the last time I took chemistry was in 1968, and I wasn't sure I had much to offer him concerning electron shells. He looked at me with genuine wonder. I realized that he thought I was the professor.

I got things straightened out with my lab partner and we worked well with each other for the rest of the term. I always felt like the odd man out with everyone, though, not just because I was older, but because I was juggling the worlds of pre-med, insurance, and family. Often those worlds collided in weird ways.

One afternoon I left my Gross Anatomy class and caught a bus downtown to put in some hours at the insurance company. I carried my homework — a half-dissected cat — with me in a bag. The bus was crowded, and I grabbed an empty seat next to a pleasant white-haired older woman. Other riders nearby were looking at me with peculiar looks on their faces. There was, after all, a discernible odor of formaldehyde seeping from my baggage. My seatmate was polite and talkative, however, and soon I had told her about my career plans and my classes.

"How interesting," she said. "Is that schoolwork in your bag?" Her nose might have twitched a little.

"Yes, it is," I said brightly. She looked like the textbook cat-lover and I really didn't want to get into unpleasant details.

"Taking your work home with you."

"Yes, ma'am!"

She wouldn't give up.

"What's *in* your bag, young man?"

"Well, it's a cat."

She turned her head toward the front of the bus and we spent an uncomfortable twenty minutes without a further word.

My juggling act was hard to manage, but I was driven now in a way I hadn't felt before. I had never needed to work very hard in school, especially in math, so I coasted through high school and my undergrad major with as little effort as possible. Someone who saw me before and after might not have believed I was the same person. Strangely enough, the professor I had in that pre-med chemistry course (the real one, not the guy in the powder-blue suit) was someone who had seen both pre- and post-Kevin. He was a judge from a high school science fair I was forced to participate in. It had been quite literally a last-minute job. By the morning of the fair the friends I had roped in and I had run out of vowels to stick on the posters. The board on the far right looked like it was in Czech. My answers to the judges' questions could have been in another language for all the sense they made. I wasn't sure if the professor had recognized me in his class. He had. I was called into his office for a conference one day.

"Mr. Kington, you're doing extremely well in this course."

"Thank you, professor," I said.

"I can't, for the life of me, understand why," he replied.

When we got talking about the science fair he said, "You were by far the most ill-prepared student I have ever judged. What happened?"

Maturity happened. That and I found a sense of mission that I never possessed before. Luckily for me, like most travelers at the start of a quest, I didn't know how long it would take or how difficult it would be.

I began those pre-med science courses in September of 1978 and I finished them in 1980. It took another year to get into med school. Before that happened, though, I needed more money than I was making at the insurance company, so I had a series of odd jobs in every sense of the term. I was a waiter at a ritzy country club and a computer programmer for all sorts of people. I still wasn't making enough. I went to an ancient device called the Yellow Pages and started cold-calling all the companies listed under data processing. I told whoever was willing to listen that I was getting ready to start medical school and I needed a part-time job. The responses were not enthusiastic. Eventually I got someone who did listen, but all he said was,

"Didn't I just talk to you about twenty minutes ago?"

"Well, are you listed in the Yellow Pages under two different names?"

He started laughing and said, "That's what you're doing? You're calling everyone listed in the Yellow Pages?"

"Yep," I said, "Do you have a better idea?"

So he laughed again and said, "Now you've got me intrigued. I want to talk to you. Why don't you meet me down at Frisch's on campus this Saturday?"

On a pretty fall morning at 10:00, I went down to Frisch's restaurant. It was a football Saturday, and the place was crowded. I'm looking for a fifty-year-old gentleman with gray hair when a chubby, thirtyish guy in black hornrims and a red Ohio State sweatshirt walks up to me and says,

"Are you Kevin? I'm Larry. Don's not going to be here for a while, so he asked me to meet with you and talk to you."

We sat at a booth in the diner and talked about football. Then about football. Finally, about football. At some point Don showed up, casually elegant in a Brooks Brothers jacket and no tie. He gave me a strong handshake and turned to Larry,

"What do you think, kid? Can he do the job?"

Larry said "Oh, absolutely!"

"Great," Don said, "Then we don't need to talk about work. Let's talk about football."

He told me to come down to the office, get a computer, take it home, and start working. So that was that. When he was getting into his car I realized that I hadn't asked him how much I would make just as he turned to me and said,

"Kevin, you never asked me how much you wanted to make."

I thought this was my chance; I would shoot for the moon, 1981-style. I said I thought I should make $12.50 an hour. Don agreed. Then the door closed, and his Cadillac zoomed away. I stood there in the middle of the parking lot thinking, "Damn. I should have asked for twenty bucks."

So now I was working for the insurance company downtown and for Don at home. I was spending a lot of time in my basement doing payroll records on a terminal that gave me three hundred words a minute. Three hundred baud. Consider that, computer geeks. I'd give it a print command and I'd go make a sandwich. I had time to make a big one. I'd come back and watch the screen while the machine was still printing. I began to wonder how many hours I should bill for since much of my time was spent chewing and listening to the printer. My conscience was bothering me, so

I thought I'd bill for just half the hours I was spending. And I didn't want to get fired for taking too long.

I went into Don's office and I showed him what I'd done and told him it took me three hours to do it. I found out later that he was flabbergasted. He thought it would take me around fifteen hours. So he gave me another project and as I was walking out of his office a small miracle happened.

I looked in another room and there were two guys in there in their forties or fifties — pretty old for programmers back in those days. They were an odd pair. One was over six feet tall, gaunt as a runner and neatly dressed. The other was short, heavy, and a shirttail was trying to escape. They were cranked up about something, pointing and arguing, and I was curious, so I stepped in. Taped to three walls was a printout that looked like gibberish, but after a closer look I could tell what it was — hexadecimal, which is a base-sixteen computer code. It was an insurance master file, something that maybe a few hundred people in the country were familiar with and I, because of my actuarial work, was one of those people.

Don had just gotten a big contract with an insurance company and they had sent his staff the master file. They were having a hell of a time trying to figure it out — riffling through manuals, poring over the huge sheets.

I said, "What are you guys doing?" They looked at me like I was some idiot kid.

"Well, we got this master file from an insurance company in Texas and we're trying to read it. We've got these manuals that tell us the format."

"Oh, yeah," I said, "It's in hexadecimal."

They raised their eyebrows and said that it was, indeed, in hexadecimal. I strolled up to the sheet and told them that I could read a bit of hexadecimal. "What's this M here?" I asked. "And here's a D. Hmmm." I knew the answer to all my questions, of course, but I put on a great act of casually working out the code.

They said, in a dazed way, "The M stands for master record. That's the start of a file."

"Oh. Okay. There's a number right after it. That must be the length of the file, huh? 1,126. That's a pretty long record. If we follow that over here we'll find the end of the file. Yep. Here's another M."

Now they were getting interested. I started circling fields with my pen and they were going crazy. I said, "Yeah, I see what you're doing. Very cool." And I walked out. They went running into Don's office.

"Who was that guy?"

"That's just Kevin," Don said. "He's doing some part-time work for us."

"Well, you've got to hire him. He knows how to read hexadecimal and he knows how to read our insurance master file. He just walked in here and started reading it to us."

Don called me and asked me what it would take to get me to quit all my other work and come to work full-time for him. I wasn't going to make the same mistake I'd made before. I said, "Gee, they've been so good to me at the insurance company. I don't know if I could quit. They've been so loyal while I've been getting ready for med school."

He said, "Yeah, yeah, yeah. How much would you like to make?"

I said, "Well, I need to make enough for med school, so I'd want twenty dollars an hour and no limit on the number of hours I could bill for. And I also would like my income deferred — half of it now and half after I start med school."

Don said, "Give them your two weeks' notice."

I felt like I was jumping off a cliff. The insurance company had been my security blanket, the last tie to my old life. Gulp.

Chapter 2

Watch That First Step

In Which I Try to Act Like My Kid with Mixed Results

I started medical school in the fall of 1981 and something was wrong. I had been sleeping badly for a couple of weeks, waking in the dark and lying there. My appetite was shot. I was losing weight. What a great time to be getting sick, I told myself. I wasn't used to such feelings, but the first morning of classes I recognized the obvious. I thought I had been excited about school, but I was terrified. On a Monday morning in late September on my way to class, I dropped my eight-year-old son at his school right across from the campus. Tim had chatted away happily in the car about how much he liked his subjects and his teacher, then ran for the schoolhouse so quickly that I had to lean over and pull his door shut. I headed for the parking garage near the med school feeling like Louis XVI going to the guillotine. And Louis didn't have to find a parking spot. When I thought about Tim's behavior, the role reversal was embarrassing.

In fact, they did their best to scare us on that first day — giving us the old "look around you" routine during our orientation. "Look to your left. Now look to your right. In a year, only one of you will still be here." Well, that wasn't really true. If you screwed up a course and were willing to retake it, they let you. There was a guy in my class who had been in med school for seven years. He was maybe the worst student in the history of that large and venerable institution. He made up for his shortcomings with persistence, though, and finally graduated when I did. I've always liked the med school gag that goes "What do you call the person who graduates last in his class?" The answer, of course, is "Doctor." In any case, this guy ended up in L.A. as one of those doctors to the stars. Stubbornness has its rewards, I guess.

Just because they exaggerated the attrition rate of med school doesn't mean they exaggerated its difficulty. It was grueling, and a lot of people did quit. We took the standard scientific mix of labs and lectures, but the lectures were very long and very detailed. I had never taken so many notes in my life. I have a theory that the legendarily bad handwriting of doctors is the result of years of relentless note-taking.

We were able to slow the flow from the fire hose a bit by using note services. Students would record lectures and share the tapes. If you missed a definition, explanation, or class, it wasn't a disaster. Sometimes students would come in, turn on the tape recorder and head off to do one of the other endless tasks in their workload. Some of the teachers were not amused by the practice. A friend of mine once came in to retrieve his recorder from a classroom and found the prof's tape recorder on the lectern lecturing to a dozen other tape recorders.

Through the blur of work and study during that first year it's the memories of those professors that stand out most strongly. One, my anatomy teacher Jan Negulesco, was an artist in every sense of the word. There are plenty of people in medicine who like to think that they know it all. This guy really did. You couldn't stump him on a point of anatomy. He could ID anything. That may not sound amazing, but it truly is. Professors are supposed to know their field, of course. Consider, though, that not everyone's organs look alike. They aren't always the same size. They aren't always in the same place. Disease may alter their appearance. So can the clumsy scalpels of medical students. Negulesco always knew what you were looking at. Always. And he could draw like da Vinci. When we walked into his classroom he had everything we would be looking at that day up on the board in colored chalk and it was impressive — complete, detailed, and gracefully artistic. There were three anatomy professors in the school. They were all good, and each class thought that they had the best one. It was like being in a fraternity or sorority. I'm pretty sure I had the best.

They didn't expect us to draw like Negulesco, but we did have a book of anatomical sketches that we were asked to fill in accurately with colored pencils. Yes, an anatomy coloring book. Actually it was very useful, but it nearly got me in trouble. I had brought some of the pages home with me to fill in and had left them lying around. My six-year-old daughter and a friend found them and saw that they were perfect for coloring. Nancy caught the neighbor girl going out the door with some loose sheets of paper and grabbed them at the last moment. They were highly detailed illustrations of the female genital and rectal areas. The kid's Christian fundamentalist mother just missed changing her mind about those nice Kingtons.

Along with the various anatomical illustrations I also got a cadaver that I shared with five other students. We called ours Rudy in honor of one of our fellow students who was a little odd — or maybe I should say slightly odder than the rest of us. (The name just rhymed with hers, by the way. We were sarcastic, not cruel.) Another cadaver that had emphysema was Wheezer. Rudy was the only one of the cadavers in our class that had a uterus; the other female cadavers had all had hysterectomies. So we shared Rudy when we got to that section of the course. Two of the students in our group became gynecologists. Whether it was because of the luck of the draw in getting Rudy I've never been sure. We kept our cadavers all year as we worked through every system. Despite whatever irreverence that we showed toward them, they were the greatest learning tool that we had and we appreciated it. In fact, the irreverence might have been a way to give us a little emotional distance from the reality that not long ago these had been living human beings with their own emotions, joys, and fears.

Medical school begins with two years of classes and labs where you learn the material and finishes with two years of clinical work in a hospital where you put what you learned into practice. The anatomy course resembled the hospital clinical courses because it was so hands-on. The nasty catch-22 is that when you first start dissecting you don't know what the hell you're doing but because of simple practicality you're forced to begin with one of the most difficult systems — the skin, muscles, and nerves of the back. You're dealing with some of the most delicate parts of the human body when your dissection skills are the worst they'll ever be. By the end of the third week you are completely convinced that you're a terrible medical student. Little by little, though, your hand gets steadier and your eye gets better. We dissected and dissected and dissected and the suffocating, pickle-like smell of formaldehyde stayed on us for much of that first year.

The anatomy, physiology, and biochemistry courses lasted both semesters of the first year as we learned the parts of the body, how they interacted, and what made them function. Filling out that year and the second were lectures by specialists who rotated through our lecture hall with varying degrees of effectiveness. One of the most memorable guys was William Havener, the head of ophthalmology. Dr. Havener had been around forever and was something of a legend. The university's eye institute is now named after him. He always started his initial lecture by asking, "Who knows what the most important square inch of the body is?"

Well, most med students are smart enough to know that the answer for an ophthalmologist is probably going to be the eye.

Then he would ask, "If your Aunt Millie passes out in front of you what should you do?"

A number of useful answers might occur to you in this case, but the right one was, "You need to look in her eye." We all laughed about that one.

Then one day he was giving a lecture about the use of atropine, which is used to dilate the pupils so that you can examine the eye. He passed around a bottle of the stuff and it got to Tim Wilson, an extremely bright and extremely hyper student. Tim started fiddling with the bottle.

"I want you to be very careful with that bottle," Havener said, "There's enough atropine in there to poison everyone in this city."

Tim looked shaken. He might have had the lid off; I couldn't see. He stood up quickly, stepped onto the stage to give the bottle back to Havener and, in a very stage worthy way, passed out and dropped to the floor. I never found out whether it was because of the atropine or because he was just an intense guy. Poor Tim was sprawled out on the stage and Havener, by God, knelt down beside him, pulled back his eyelids and looked in his eye. Then he told one of us to call the ER, which was right next door, and after waiting for about thirty seconds started his lecture again — pacing the stage and carefully stepping over Tim each time. The squad got there in a few minutes, strapped Tim to a stretcher and hauled him off.

"I suppose," Havener said to us, "that because of today's distraction, I'll give the class the option of continuing with the lecture or going home now." The room was empty in about ten seconds.

I will always admire Dr. Havener for being a practitioner of what he preached. He was also a pretty good lecturer. Not all of the docs were. One was so unbearably bad that it became rather tragic. Dr. Blank, as I'll call him, didn't really lecture. He read. He read in a slow, monotonous, relentless voice. I won't mention his specialty. In a just world he would have been an anesthesiologist.

After a few weeks of his lectures a couple of the more impatient students got the bright idea of pieing him. They put on greasepaint, dressed up like clowns, walked onto the stage, shoved a pie in his face and ran out of the hall. It was awful. If they thought that the class would find it funny they were wrong. There was a little bit of surprised laughter, but mostly there were gasps. Blank was devastated. The lecture was over, of course, and the next day he quietly told us how humiliated and hurt he was. It really was hard to listen to. They never caught the students who did it, though there was an investigation and the dean offered a reward. For me, it was an object lesson in the importance of paying respect even where it might not seem to be due. It's also one of the most remarkable examples of that large topic How Very Smart People Can Do Very Dumb Things.

Another of our lecturers, Leopold Liss, spoke to us about his research on Alzheimer's disease. That was a little odd for me, because Dr. Liss and I had lived in the same neighborhood when I was young and we kids had thought he was quite a scary character. He had wild-looking, white Einstein hair and when we saw him driving his Volvo we'd whisper to each other, "He operates on dead people's brains!" How that got into the neighborhood folklore I have no idea, but it turned out to be perfectly true. As a pathologist studying Alzheimer's, Liss did indeed operate on dead people's brains. He wasn't scary, though, he was brilliant and articulate. (Dr. Liss's son, Dick, had gone to my high school. He was a very prominent student and when, every so often, "Dick Liss" would get read over the intercom hilarity ensued. That was only among the less mature students, of course.)

Our lecturers assigned textbook chapters and early on I discovered a disturbing reality about medical school. There was no way to do all the reading. I prided myself on being a very quick reader with a very good memory, but I could work steadily for ten or twelve hours a day and still not get through half the assignment. The other students had the same experience. Just as our note services helped us with lecture material, we formed study groups to help with the reading. Ultimately, though, mastering all of it was an impossible job, so you just began to get a feel for what you could ignore. It was a peculiar way to teach, I thought.

Thirty years later I still have questions about some of the teaching methods medical schools employ. The sheer volume of information thrown at us sometimes felt more like initiation than education. "I had to do it, so you do, too." One of our many texts was *The Nail*, 1,700 pages about the fingernail. A medical education certainly has to be broad and deep, but obscurity is obscurity. Some of the things we learned I've never come close to using. Take the Krebs Cycle, for instance. It describes at great length and endless terminology how we turn food into energy — important stuff for a biochemist, certainly, but in the many years since I memorized it I haven't had to use the information once. (However, if I ever encounter a patient who can't synthesize citrulline I'll know to feed him watermelon.) It seems to me that having to study things that are irrelevant uses a lot of time that could be spent studying things that are important.

That initiation process runs deeply through the structure and customs of med school and I've thought many times that there's a clear parallel between a medical education and hazing rituals. Great mental stress is administered, in many cases just for the sake of it, and the physical demands of a residency are terrible. Moreover, like hazing, the habits are perpetuated by those who were abused. Studies have been done on how hard residents work and how little they sleep. There's a real correlation between the number of hours worked and the number of medical mistakes made, but there's also huge resistance to cutting work hours from doctors of my generation. "These new residents," you'll hear, "don't want to work more than eighty hours a week." Workloads have been lightened a little, but new doctors are still worked beyond exhaustion. "I had to do it, so you do, too."

An alternative offered to the lecture/discussion track was independent study, and if I had had any brains when I began med school I would have done that. I was afraid, though, that I wouldn't have the discipline to work independently and that the distractions of the family would get in the way. For all of its shortcomings, taking the lecture route did let me get to know my fellow students and work with them in a way I wouldn't have been able to do on the independent study track.

They were a group of very bright, driven, and quirky people. I wasn't the oldest. There was a guy, Warren McCay, who had been teaching high school chemistry and had three kids. He was about six or seven years older than I was. I wasn't the tallest. That was Rob Phelps. He was six foot nine and had played basketball in college. The best athlete was Joe Terry, who had played football at Harvard. I have many lifelong friends from those years and I'm still in touch with most of them. Along with Nancy and the kids they were the ones who helped keep me sane and centered.

Jeff Stockfish, who became an ophthalmologist, always sat with me in the back of the lecture hall. We'd do the crossword in the student newspaper every morning and watch our fellow students. It could be quite a show. There was one guy who was a mystery. He came in about ten minutes late every day, sprinted down the steps two at a time, found a desk, put his head down and promptly fell asleep. So Jeff and I would do our crossword, listen to the lectures, and when they were over we'd wake him up and he'd go home. We used to make up stories about what he was doing outside the classroom. We knew that he must be very busy, because he certainly was always late and tired. One of our fantasies was that he was making recombinant DNA in his garage, and it turned out that that wasn't too far from the truth. He worked in a genetics lab on campus, and he was one of the smartest people in our program. He had to be, considering that he heard nearly none of the lectures that he attended. He must have had a very good study group and an even better memory.

The real go-getters sat right in front, as they always do. Tim Wilson sat there. That's how he ended up with Dr. Havener's bottle of atropine. There was a young woman who was among the brightest of us and certainly the luckiest. During one of Havener's lectures on the eye he put a slide of a retina up on the screen and said, "If any of you can tell me the diagnosis here, I will give you a residency in ophthalmology."

That woman's hand shot up in a second and she came up with a diagnosis that the rest of us had never even heard of. Havener was dumbfounded. "That's correct! Are you interested in a residency in ophthalmology?"

She said, "I sure am."

He had her come up on stage, got her name, and she ended up with a residency right there.

We had our failures, too. One of our worst students always took notes in calligraphy. What a weird choice. He was a wonderful calligrapher, and his notebook was beautiful. The problem was that it wasn't very big. When a lecturer is loading you up with case studies and involved terminology at high speed, calligraphy just isn't a good option. There's no doubt that that guy had the prettiest set of notes in our or anyone else's medical school, but he was there for a very, very long time.

One of our best students became one of the worst. Geno had been a shark at the beginning of our coursework. He always finished his tests ahead of everyone and made sure that you knew about his Mensa membership. Then his girlfriend left him, and he fell apart. He still made a point of finishing his tests first, but now the answers were wrong. His grades plummeted, and he was a mess for most of our second year.

He pulled out of his tailspin, but it was a demonstration to me of how intelligence is not the only factor in med school success. Your emotional attitude plays just as big a part. It also brought home to me just how lucky I was in that respect. Nancy was a saint throughout med school and, later, my residency. She listened to my complaints and worries about school, gave me advice, and ran the house with efficiency and generosity. I never had to cook, clean, shop for groceries, birthdays, or Christmas. The stability that gave me was a big reason that I was able to succeed. The kids turned out to be a big help, too. They were one, three, five, and seven when I started med school and one, three, five, seven, and nine in my third year when I did my pediatric rotation. So I had the double advantage of being an expert in childhood development and a veteran of the "kiddy crud" that laid low many of my younger classmates. They were sick at least a fourth of their pediatric rotation, and I had already suffered through all the childhood diseases. Most importantly, by the time I got through that second year I realized that I could do the work and that I could become, eventually, a good doctor. It would be years before I began to be able to see in the way a good doctor must, but thanks to Nancy, the kids, my friends (and a movie) I was on my way and I felt it. The third year was the beginning of clinical work, though, and my fledgling confidence was going to be put to the test again.

Chapter 3

Admitted to the Hospital

*In Which I Begin to Look Like a Doctor
While Knowing Very Little*

The beginning of clinical work is the point where you move from the classroom to the hospital and begin working under your teachers. Now they're no longer larger than life figures speaking to you from behind a lectern; they're larger than life figures telling you to get the lead out and get to work. The student moves through two-month rotations in different specialties: psychiatry, pediatrics, obstetrics-gynecology, surgery, and internal medicine. It's a sort of matchmaking process. Ideally, students find a specialty that matches their interests and abilities, or they find out if the medical field they've been interested in is a good fit.

My original interest had been psychiatry, and I felt fortunate that that was my first rotation. The director of the section was Thomas Szabo, a very interesting guy. Szabo and his wife had made it through the Hungarian Iron Curtain in a particularly brazen and gutty way — dressing up in wedding clothes, sneaking across the border between armed guard towers, and accompanying the guests at a wedding ceremony. They just left the church and kept going.

Szabo was an enthusiastic disciple of psychiatry, but it didn't take me long to realize that my enthusiasm was limited. One of my first assignments was doing a history and physical on a young woman who had attempted suicide. When I entered the exam room she was curled up in a chair pushed into the far corner of the room.

"Hello, I'm Dr. Kington and I'm here to ask you some questions and do a physical examination."

"You're no doctor!" she said with a disturbing amount of energy.

Hey, no problem. I had been schooled on what to say if anyone questioned my measly credentials.

"Well, it's true that I'm not an M.D. yet, but I am a student doctor."

"No! You're not a doctor!"

I went to Szabo and told him that it was going badly, and he told me that if I let every patient I interviewed run the interview process I'd be a damn bad psychiatrist. So I went back and told the young woman that we could skip the physical, but I really would appreciate it if she'd answer a few questions. She reluctantly agreed and as I worked with her over the next couple of days she began to trust me. She even let me do the physical.

Then one afternoon while I was talking with her she looked at me and said, "Kevin, when did you become a doctor? I thought you were an actuary."

My God! She knew me from the insurance company! She was absolutely right to believe that I wasn't a doctor. Just because you're paranoid doesn't mean you're wrong.

Another memorable case was a catatonic patient with textbook symptoms. She stared dead-eyed with no recognition or reaction. If you raised her arm it stayed there. It was disturbing to see a patient so apparently beyond help, but Szabo was optimistic.

"We're going to do shock treatment tomorrow. You won't believe it's the same woman after that."

"You're still performing shock treatment? I thought that wasn't even done anymore."

He laughed. "It still has its place. Get here tomorrow. You'll be surprised."

I did get there in time to catch Szabo in the hall after the procedure.

"Well, Kington, she's talking up a storm."

I could hardly believe him, but he grabbed my arm and pulled me into the patient's room and yes, by golly, she was talking. In fact, she was arguing loudly with someone I couldn't see.

"Dr. Szabo, she seems to be having an argument with the devil."

"Yes, isn't it wonderful? Yesterday she was fully catatonic and now she's talking and talking."

It began to dawn on me then that if getting a patient to the point of yelling at the devil is considered a great improvement psychiatry might not be my field. Qualified victories and long-term maintenance of chronic conditions weren't my style. I had the same feeling in my renal rotation. A lot of patients with kidney failure are there because of something they've done — alcoholism, drug addiction, non-compliant diabetes — and that can involve guilt, blame, and family problems. Even without those issues, kidney failure is a difficult, intractable condition. The patients' personal struggles meant that a lot of them didn't handle their dialysis schedules well, so they came into the hospital in a coma. Then the med student was responsible for their history and physical.

So my first day on renal I had six spinal taps to do, which are difficult and time-consuming, and I had three history and physicals on patients in comas. A resident had shown me how to do the spinal tap, better known to doctors as a lumbar puncture. You insert a needle into the canal that surrounds the spine and draw out some of the fluid that bathes it. The needle slides in between a couple of lumbar bones or vertebrae. That's in theory. In reality, some vertebrae are in bad shape, and it's hard for the inexperienced to find an insertion point and make sure the needle stays in that canal. The spinal tap has a reputation for being painful. It certainly was for me.

And if you've never taken a medical history from a patient in a coma you really haven't lived. How do you do that? You read all the previous records and histories on the patient and then try to reconstruct what has happened since then by looking at what condition the patient is in now. You're expected, in other words, to be Sherlock Holmes. My renal attending had gone through many med students who had told him that they couldn't take a history because the patient was unconscious; the attending did not accept that as an answer.

I very much wanted to change the lives of patients for the better, and sometimes I felt as mired in those stubborn conditions as they did. After the psychiatry and renal rotations it became clear to me that I liked decisive actions that made an immediate improvement. I liked surgery.

Surgeons are well-known, perhaps notorious, for decisiveness. "Bang, bang," goes the surgeon in the joke, "Was that a duck?"

Bill Gary, the chairman of the Department of Surgery, was the archetypal surgeon: silver-haired, handsome, and very, very sure of himself. He also was brutally sarcastic. He led what was called an M and M session — morbidity and mortality — that allowed residents to review cases that resulted in death or damage to the patient. It's crucial to review procedures that have failed, but Gary ran the session like a bullring, and you sure didn't want to be the one who got gored. Dozens of doctors gathered to ask a first- or second-year resident questions about a bad outcome. One hapless resident had lost a patient whose blood pressure sank to a fatal level. It had been dangerously high, and the resident wrote an order for a drug called Apresoline to lower it. The drug order, though, wasn't flexible enough to allow the nurses to adjust the frequency as the drug began to work. So the final dose was given when the patient's blood pressure was only 90 over 60. Gary was scathing.

"Doctor, I think we all know the ABCs of resuscitation here. We just never knew that the A stood for Apresoline."

Gary had a great reputation as a surgeon, but even the other surgeons thought he was a bit, well, overconfident. Two of my favorite guys to work with, Dan Barnes and Nick Howe, both outstanding operators, once ran into an odd-looking growth on a liver while the patient was open. They weren't sure what it was and since Gary was operating next door they asked him over to take a look. He came over and told them it was just a benign pedunculated tumor (one on a stem).

"It'll shell right out of there," he said, "Want me to come over when I'm finished and do it for you?"

They accepted his offer, but while he was gone they ordered in multiple units of blood. They admired Gary, but they wanted to be on the safe side of that bulletproof confidence.

Gary came in, took a scalpel, whacked the stem of the tumor right off, and there was a geyser of blood. It looked like an episode of MASH. Dan and Nick, superb technicians that they were, feverishly started to clamp and tie off spraying arteries. They used to brag to each other (and anyone else within earshot) about who could tie off faster and they used every bit of their considerable skill on this patient. I counted forty-three arteries tied in under three minutes.

"See, I told you it would shell right out of there," Gary said as he walked out of the OR

There was also John Henry Walton, whose specialty was oncology. He had been the first surgeon I met in my surgical rotation. I thought of cancer surgery as a tragic specialty and didn't want to face the stress of it, so I put that choice last on my rotation list. I got it first, of course. Walton was famous for being a screamer. He would vent his spleen at full volume in the operating room at anyone who happened to be there.

"Nurse, are you on vacation? Get me that clamp!"

"Somebody *help* the doctor!"

"This patient is in major hemorrhage!" (The patient was actually bleeding rather normally.)

Once I didn't move quickly enough and he yelled, "Nurse, get me a gun. This medical student is too stupid to live." I didn't know it then, but it was one of his favorite lines. He used it again on another student toward the end of my rotation and a nurse, who had heard it too many times, left the operating table and returned with a squirt gun on a tray. Without missing a beat, he picked it up, squirted the student in the chest three times, returned it to the tray and went back to work.

Walton could be a pain in the ass, but he was a fine surgeon with meticulous standards. Woe be the resident or med student who didn't meet them. It was quite something, then, to watch Walton collide with The World's Worst Intern. The WWI was a Saudi who, we med students figured, must have been a prince whose father endowed a hospital wing. Considering his competence there was no other explanation for his presence. He earned his nickname the old-fashioned way, by doing virtually nothing whenever humanly possible. His trademarked expression was "No problem."

"Doctor, did you do a history and physical on the new patient?"

"No problem!"

Once you had worked a little with this guy you came to realize that "no problem" did not mean that the H and P had been done; it meant that it hadn't been done and he didn't think that was a problem. Before I witnessed Walton's legendary run-in with the World's Worst Intern I thought I had heard him scream before. Those had just been affectionate whispers.

Seven of us, including Dr. Walton, me, and the WWI had scrubbed to operate on a patient with esophageal cancer, and as Walton was drying his hands in the scrub room he began moving his head strangely and squinting through the glass into the OR where the patient lay ready on the operating table.

"What is *that*?!"

We all went to the window and looked in. The patient was being prepped and on her left breast there was a huge, dark, fungating mass. We could see it easily from across the room. Walton exploded.

"Goddamn it! Goddamn it, where's this woman's chart? Open her chart!"

So I had to break scrub, brought him her chart, and opened it up to the H and P. It said Breasts: No masses or discharge. It was written in a scribble that looked very much like someone rushing through an exam. The intern obviously had never looked at this patient's breasts. So Walton went into the OR and said something that today you could never say.

"Okay, after we're done with her esophagus we're going to do a double mastectomy."

The nurse said, "Doctor, the patient's already asleep."

He said, "I know. She'll thank me for it later."

Rules for patient consent have changed since then, I'm happy to say. Walton certainly had her welfare in mind, though. We knew she was a cancer patient, and this was rather clearly an advanced malignancy. There was no time to waste and she hardly needed a second round of anesthesia.

So he did both an esophageal reanastomosis and, with no consent, a double mastectomy, and when he was done and we were cleaned up, he ordered all of us into a stairwell on the 11th floor. Here were the World's Worst Intern, a chief resident, four medical students of varying degrees of talent, and Walton. Then he began screaming at us. He continued screaming for about forty-five minutes. Subjects, among a great many, included our intelligence, our ethics, our work habits, our medical futures, and our ancestry. Finally, he went up to each medical student, got a few inches from his face, and repeated the same thing. "You will examine *every* limb and *every* aperture of *every* patient *every* day. Or you will come to me and tell me that you don't want to do that and that will be just fine with me. Because then … You. Will. Get. The. Box."

Getting the box! The medical professor's kiss of death. At the bottom of every student's grade report was a sentence that read: This student did not complete this rotation, and next to it was a small box. Having that box ticked was worse than any F grade.

Walton liked using the box as a threat: "Kington, tell me the only two reasons not to do a digital rectal exam on a patient."

"Uh, no finger or no rectum?"

"Precisely. Any other answer gets you the box."

It's too bad that there wasn't a box to tick for interns. I lost track of the WWI, but I can't imagine him faring very well professionally after that. Walton was a prestigious surgeon whose opinion carried weight and he knew whose scrawl was on that H and P. The screaming session in the stairwell became famous. It was heard all the way down on the first floor of the hospital and I fielded questions about it for days.

Walton and I became closer as time went on. He was a complicated man: hot-tempered and dictatorial, but extremely skilled — a good teacher with an amazingly huge ego. He had a pet theory, which got some press coverage in the 70s and which has since been disproved, that caffeine use was a precursor to fibrocystic breast disease. I operated with him once and later he was sitting in the recovery room writing his orders. He turned to me and said, "Kington, when I'm famous you can say you knew me when. I'm twenty years ahead of my time. I'm published in all the journals. No one believes me yet, but time will tell."

I had no idea that his theory had been taken that seriously.

I said, "You're published in all the journals?"

"Yes," he answered. "*Ladies Home Journal*; *Good Housekeeping*; *Redbook*. All of them."

We got some fun out of awarding the WWI his title, but a chilling reality we weren't aware of was that there was another intern in that year's class who was beyond any designation of bad. He was a psychopath: the serial killer Michael Swango. Swango ended up murdering dozens of patients, and he might have begun his killing career at our hospital. He was a neurosurgery intern and all the med students thought he was a little weird. In fact, Swango had asked out one of my classmates, but she was wise enough to decline.

Swango sometimes asked you for the potassium level on a patient and if you didn't know it he'd make you hit the floor and give him twenty pushups. He had come from the military and that was his way of reminding you. It was also a way, I think, of demeaning you and exercising, in a tiny way, whatever cruel instincts dwell in the mind of a killer.

When we med students started our rounds in the morning and a bed was made with no occupant we'd say that the patient had "Swangoed." That's how close we were to catching on to him. We just never made that jump from sarcastic dismissal of his skills to the realization of what he really was.

Finally, the roommate of a victim saw Swango inject a patient with something and leave. A minute later the patient went into a seizure. The nurses called a code and when the code team came Swango followed them in and, according to the witness, stood in the doorway and watched with a little smirk on his face. That story made it to the dean and resulted in an investigation. After that Swango was always visually supervised and his contract wasn't renewed after the internship. The university didn't call the police as they should have, though. A book was written about the situation called *Blind Eye: How the Medical Establishment Let a Doctor Get Away with Murder* by James B. Stewart (New York City: Simon and Schuster, 2000). It was years later, after disinterring some bodies, that the university finally realized that he might have killed seven patients there. Tragically, Swango continued his medical career, kept a step ahead of the law, and ended up killing many more people on a couple of continents before he was arrested and jailed.

Once Swango was in jail, a former classmate wrote a letter to the friend of ours that Swango had tried to date. He asked her if she would be his prison pen pal and signed Swango's name. She was pretty upset about it for a day or so until he told her he had written it. Even she found it funny — eventually.

I worked under Gary and Walton during my general surgery rotation, then that was followed by two-week assignments in different surgical subspecialties. My most memorable were plastic and orthopedic surgery. It was in plastic surgery that I finally learned how to tie a knot, and it was a crash course. When I walked into the OR on my first day there were two residents working on a patient whose leg had been amputated. They were transferring part of a back muscle, the latissimus dorsi, to the stump of the patient's leg, and to do that they had removed the entire muscle. The latissimus dorsi is a big, triangular muscle — the largest one in the body. When it's missing you definitely notice it. Attaching a flap of the muscle to the leg involved microsurgery, so they were down near the knee with their microscopes and one of them looked up and said, "Good. You're here. You're late. Close that wound in the back."

I looked down at the Grand Canyon. This was a big guy in the first place and there was a hole in his back that was probably two feet by one-and-a-half feet. I had never tied a knot in surgery. So I said, "You'd better show me how to start."

One of the surgeons got up disgustedly from his microscope, came over, threw a suture and tied it down and said,

"Just do this over and over again; sew it at the bottom and gradually it'll close."

So I started. This was about 8:00 in the morning. I sewed and I sewed and I sewed. After about fifty or sixty stitches I really felt like I was getting the hang of it. Unfortunately, I had closed only a few inches of the massive wound, and I really was afraid of those surgeons stepping up and seeing how little work I'd gotten done. After all those stitches it still looked like the Grand Canyon. I was sweating, worrying, sewing, and pretty soon I didn't even know what my hands were doing. It was automatic. Then the dreaded moment came when the resident got up, walked over and said, "Let's see how you're doing."

He looked down at the back and said, "Well, we've still got another six hours on the knee. Do you want to take a break for lunch?"

Wow. I had no idea microsurgery could take that long. So I went to lunch. Once I knew I had six hours to get the wound closed I stopped worrying. It took me the whole six hours, though, to close that back, and I ended up doing thousands of stitches. After that case I most definitely knew how to tie knots.

While plastic surgery could be that sort of meticulous, small-scale procedure, orthopedic surgery was its bizarre opposite. It's like no other kind of surgery; really it's more like carpentry. Orthopedists use screws, hammers, and chisels, and there's a lot of pounding. The first day I came into the OR one of the orthopedists looked at me and said, "Oh, good! A big guy." They had me holding the patient with his leg up over my shoulder for three hours, and he was another big guy, with a big, thick leg. That would have been hard enough, but they also put me in a spacesuit that draws the air off you and takes it, and all your germs, out of the room. It was pretty hot in there. I was standing for three hours holding this 300-pound man's leg up in the air. So my first view of orthopedic surgery was through the foggy window of an astronaut suit with sweat pouring down into its unseen nether regions. I made my decision about an orthopedic specialty that first day.

Of all the surgeons I met on my rotation, either in general surgery or the subspecialties, the one who gave me the greatest lesson was Big Ed Fields, an oncologist. It was with him that I first saw that central skill of the good physician — the simple, yet crucial ability to see what's in front of you. Big Ed was gruff — no nonsense, as the euphemism puts it. We had a patient with gastro-intestinal pain and suspected a tumor. Big Ed scheduled a colonoscopy which he described to me with characteristic force.

"Yeah, I scoped him. Cancer. I could see it up there. We'll go in Friday. We need to get that sucker outta there."

I was impressed and a little surprised that he could diagnose a malignancy with such confidence through just the colonoscopy image. He had done a biopsy, of course, and the results weren't back yet. But he was sure. Then the results came back, and I was the one who picked them up. The lab report read "benign tissue."

I was relieved and a little proud of myself. I would save this impressive surgeon from making a terrible mistake.

"I don't care what the lab says," Big Ed said to me when I told him, "It's cancer. We're going in."

"But, Doctor ..."

No dice. Big Ed had looked, thought it was cancer, and was operating. On Friday we scrubbed, went in, removed the growth, and the whole mass was biopsied again. It was cancer.

Lab results aren't always right. Big Ed had learned that. He also had learned to look with more than just his eyes. He looked at that mass and was sure it was malignant, then put that together with the patient's symptoms and condition and got the right conclusion, lab results be damned. That impressed me. That was where I wanted to be but wouldn't be for a very long time.

Yes, I liked surgery, but I had to admit that I didn't much care for surgeons. It wasn't a matter of getting skewered with a comment, or screamed at, or even shot at with a squirt gun. There was simply a surgeon's machismo that rubbed me the wrong way, a personality that didn't mesh well with mine. Then I did my obstetrics-gynecology rotation and I knew I was home. Ob-gyns do surgery; many of the procedures are the same (though a surgeon probably would disagree). Decisiveness is important, and results are quick. Ob-gyns, though, are far more laid back than any surgeon I ever met. I also discovered that I love delivering babies. Who wouldn't be touched by bringing a new life into the world? Who wouldn't want to be with a patient at one of the happiest moments of her life? It's even better when you can turn a potential tragedy into one of those happy moments.

I remember the first birth in my ob-gyn rotation. A third-year resident, Tom Campbell, delivered the baby. Tom was a pleasure to watch — confident, fast and sure-handed. There was nothing remarkable about the case; it was a full-term vaginal delivery like thousands that have followed in my career. In that way it was perfectly symbolic. What I remember most are the feelings I had. They were surprisingly like the ones I felt when I watched Nancy deliver our first two: a bracing sense of being part of the profound process of life and pure joy that lasted for hours. I don't drink, but after scrubbing that morning I thought, "This is what champagne must feel like." I had found what I wanted to do in medicine. Nancy loved the idea. We were products of big families and wanted one ourselves. Everything fit. The journey now had a destination, but there was still a challenging fourth year to go.

Chapter 4

Match

In Which I Prepare to Be Judged

The fourth year of medical school is very different from the other three. It's still clinical, like the third year, but there's a huge evolution in the student's confidence and ability. In the third year you're pretty much treated as a scut puppy — doing a lot of leg work for the residents, but not really treating patients. You do some procedures on them and might take them down to x-ray occasionally, but your only contribution is, "Yes, Doctor." You get to know the patients and you get to know the plan, but you don't make any management decisions.

In the fourth year, though, you become a kind of sub-intern (and some rotations even use that term officially). You do H and Ps, look at charts, diagnose as well as your experience allows, and voice opinions. Those opinions are often shot down by the resident, but you're taken seriously enough to be listened to and that's a powerful educational tool. It's a wonderful thing when a resident begins to expect you to act like a resident.

There's even more to like. The fourth year includes more elective rotations. The students get to decide most of their courses based on the subspecialty that attracts them. I did two months in ob-gyn and then did some things that I wouldn't see again, but that I thought would round me out as a physician — gastrointestinal, neurology, and family practice.

The GI rotation came first, and I enjoyed it in part because of my instructor, Eugene May. May was a real character and, professionally, he had a unique setup. He was purely a consulting physician. He had no patients of his own, but only did consultations for other doctors. So every patient he saw was a procedure; he never had any long-term patients. His office was a little hole in the wall that he rarely used, so he had little office overhead. If you were a general surgeon or an internist who needed someone to do a colonoscopy you would call May. He did that all day. We were constantly driving between a couple of local hospitals. He scoped three or four people at one, then we'd hop in his van and go scope three or four more at another. On the way he'd tape-record his notes on the colonoscopies using a different accent for each patient. He had an Irish brogue, an excitable Italian, a German, and a Spanish guy.

"Sure and 'twas eight-twenty on the loveliest o' mornin's when we started this puir lad's procedure ..."

"Herr Schmidt vass complenning uff intestinal pain ..."

Why? I never asked. Maybe it was to keep him alert during a long workday. Or maybe it was to tease his stenographer. If it was to amuse his medical students, he was very successful. He never repeated an accent on one day, so it certainly separated his cases on the tape recorder. May was a great educator. He really knew his stuff and that sense of humor helped the student remember it.

During a colonoscopy on one cancer patient we began seeing something odd on the screen. It looked like the peritoneum to me — the lining of the abdominal cavity. Then May began cursing. "Do you know what that is?"

"It looks like the peritoneum," I said.

"Do you know what that means?"

"It means we're not in the colon anymore."

"That's right, Toto."

Radiation therapy had made the patient's colon wall tissue-thin and we had perforated it with the camera.

That was one of a couple of complications during the month I was with him, and I learned from both. The colonoscopy patients received Demerol, a painkiller, and Versed, a sedative, before the procedures, and May warned me about their use.

"You have to be careful with the little old ladies, because it doesn't take much of either of those to stop their breathing."

Sure enough, halfway through the month we had an elderly woman stop breathing on us and we had to do CPR until the Demerol cleared. May was prepared for it, though, and had prepared us, so his team was able to deal with the situation quickly and confidently.

My second elective was neurology, and I liked it far less than GI. It wasn't because of the people. That team of doctors was the most brilliant I had ever worked with, and they were all younger than I was. Our attending was twenty-five years old. I don't even know how you do that; you have to be Doogie Howser, I guess. Then we had a resident who was an osteopath: a doctor of Osteopathy or a DO. MDs still sometimes look down on DOs because in the nineteenth century DOs developed their own ideas about the origins of disease. These days the education of MDs and DOs is very similar, and this resident taught me that DOs are just as smart as MDs. In fact, he was the smartest resident I ever worked with.

So I really liked that rotation, but I really disliked the field. On the neurology rotation we did our rounds to see the patients, went to their doors and discussed all their symptoms. Some poor fellow would be lying in there in a coma after a stroke — immobile and not speaking — and we went over his neurological exam. From that exam we determined precisely what nerves in the brain were affected. That's how I realized those docs were so bright. They could analyze the sensory findings, the motor findings, put it all together, and tell you the square inch of the brain that had stroked. They had the CAT scan to help them, but they hardly needed it. They could put all the symptoms and test data together in a way that I'd never seen before, and it really taught me neurology. But then we shrugged and went to the next room. It was just a kind of academic exercise because so many of the patients were never going to recover. There was no treatment for neurological damage, so if you had a stroke we could send you to physical therapy, but there wasn't anything doctors could do structurally to reverse the damage. That's changed a little bit in the years since, but neurology would have been a very frustrating field for me. You're seeing all these people with terrible diseases and your role, basically, is to tell them what's happening to them and why.

Even neurosurgery had no appeal. Some neurosurgeons work on things other than the brain. They might do surgery on the back or the nerves that enter it, and that can really benefit patients. When you're working in the brain, though, too often you're simply stopping a process that's already done its damage and keeping it from getting worse. The neurology rotation was as useful as I had hoped in terms of teaching me about the brain and how it functioned, but it was a disturbing experience that I was glad to leave behind me.

The elective in your own subspecialty is really a month-long job interview. You do a rotation at a community or university hospital and it's really a way for the people there to get to know you and evaluate you as a potential resident the next year. When I did my ob-gyn rotation I really got a taste of how different academic OB is from community hospital OB. In community hospitals you find out that there are a lot of different ways to do things — some of them good, some of them not so good. You also can find out that some of your heroes have clay feet.

I decided in my community hospital rotation that there were two kinds of obstetricians: those who like women and those who don't. (This was, of course, when there were many more men practicing ob-gyn than there are now.) There were some doctors who seemed to be in the profession solely for themselves — for power, for money, but not for the patient. In my rotation there was one attending that I never saw for more than a few minutes at a time. The nurse called him when the patient was almost ready to deliver. Then he came in, put on forceps, cut an episiotomy (an incision done to ease the passage of the baby), delivered the baby, sewed up the episiotomy, and disappeared. He never spent more than ten minutes in the hospital. Most of those women could have delivered without forceps and without an episiotomy, but it made things quicker and easier for him. That was disturbing. Then there were doctors who told you that the art of medicine goes something like this: if a patient comes in for a problem you take her to surgery and you fix it, but if there are other problems you want to make sure that she comes in for a separate visit. If you solve two problems at a time you can only send one bill.

Some doctors operate on a schedule. Literally. If the patient's pushing at 5:00 in the afternoon you know she's going to get a C-section if she doesn't deliver by 7:00. Everything's on their schedule instead of the baby's schedule. I'm not saying that most doctors at community hospitals are like these bad examples. They're not. I'm at a community hospital myself. Nor am I saying that university hospitals are exemplary. The difference is that there is more leeway at a community hospital to do your own thing as far as procedures. That can be freeing for the good physician, while the one who isn't so good can take advantage of it. At a university the protocols and procedures are rigidly prescribed. Sometimes that's a good thing and sometimes that's not. Ways of doing things in a university setting can become a little inbred. Many of the teachers have graduated from that program, so the hospital has to make the effort to bring in fresh blood.

Finally, I did my family practice rotation. I liked it, but I got a taste of what it was like to sit in an office all day talking to patients. I used to think that I would like that and even imagined having a day where I would do nothing but talk with patients about the psychological issues surrounding their illness. The family practice doc disabused me of that notion. It looked to me like too much of his time was spent quarterbacking the specialists that he sent his patients to. I wanted more hands-on work than that.

Those fourth-year clinicals were extremely valuable both for what I learned about other areas of medicine and for reaffirming my commitment to ob-gyn. With my graduation approaching I was never surer of what I wanted to do. Then it was time for the next step, because the fourth year is the time that students make their applications for residencies around the country. Since Nancy and I had five kids by this time, we wanted to stay put if possible. There were three ob-gyn programs in town — two community hospitals and the university. We were encouraged to apply to a dozen programs and because there would be a lot of ob-gyn applicants for the local hospitals, I applied at some programs on the East Coast as well. Nancy's sister lived out there and if we needed to leave town at least we would still be near family. I ended up applying to just six places: the three local hospitals and three on the East Coast. Once students interviewed at their prospective hospitals, they ranked them in terms of their interest in them. On Match Day in March the choices of students were correlated with the hospitals that wanted them. If they were lucky, the new doctors started a residency at the first choice on their list.

The interview process was intimidating. I began at my own university, and the chair of Obstetrics, Fred Zimmerman, didn't make it any easier. Zimmerman was a giant in ob-gyn. He was the editor of the *Gray Journal*, the primary scientific journal in the field, and was one of the chief examiners for oral boards. So he was used to grilling even experienced physicians who were trying for board certification in their subspecialty. Zimmerman wanted the most capable students, so he put prospective residents on the spot. It was like going to see the Wizard of Oz, just without the flames and smoke. When I went into his office he was sitting behind his big desk in a rocking chair looking like a stern grandfather. He pulled out an alarm clock which also seemed rather large, put it front and center on the desk, set it, and said, "Mr. Kington, you have five minutes to convince me that you should be a resident in my program. Begin now."

I remember almost nothing of what I said to Zimmerman, but I'm sure it was boilerplate about being a hard worker, loving the field, admiring the program, wanting to work with the best, and so on. The one thing I do remember saying is that, because of my age, I felt that I was more mature and ready for responsibility than other applicants might be.

"Mr. Kington," he replied, "All of my applicants are mature."

I felt I did pretty well, but it was certainly an uncomfortable interview. Not as uncomfortable as my friend's interview for a neurology residency at a hospital he strongly disliked. With somber eyes the chief resident asked, "Why were you drawn to neurology?"

Equally somber my friend replied, "Because I like turning people into things."

Long pause as the chief continued to study him impassively, then, "You really don't want to come here, do you?"

The interviews at the two community hospitals weren't nearly as scary, in part because I wasn't as interested in them. To give myself the widest experience, I was looking for a good mix of high-risk cases and ob-gyn surgeries, and neither of these hospitals had that.

So I went out east to look at three more programs — Bay State Hospital in Springfield, Massachusetts and Hartford Hospital and St. Francis Hospital both in Hartford, Connecticut. Those interviews went well; they all asked me back to do a second interview. Something peculiar happened, though. I had ranked the hospitals after both my first and second visits and the rankings were the opposite of one another. I had put Hartford at the top the first time out. Then I went back and worked a day and I found that it was very cliquish. There were two groups of residents who were enemies, so half of any residency was going to be pleasant and half of it wasn't.

When I went back to Bay State I put on scrubs at 7:00 in the morning and we worked full-speed without a stop until 8:30 at night. We had seven C-sections, two ectopic pregnancies, and more deliveries than I can even remember. We didn't get breakfast, lunch, or dinner. The resident kept saying that it was never that busy, but it was a little bit overwhelming. I knew I'd get a lot of experience there, but I wasn't sure I could survive it. More importantly, how could I be the kind of doctor I wanted to be in that kind of crazy environment?

At St. Francis I had really liked my first interview. If Fred Zimmerman was the grandfather, Dr. Stan, the chief resident at St. Francis was the godfather: cool, competent, and impressive. He only asked me two questions. What was the score of the NFL championship game between the Cleveland Browns and the Baltimore Colts? Who were the quarterback and receiver on the Browns who did most of their scoring? Since I'm from Cleveland and am a Browns fan I knew both answers. I later found out that he asked my good friend Tony, who is from New Jersey, a question about the New York Knicks basketball team.

I think there was a method to Stanley's apparent madness. He had a pretty good idea of who we were academically and was probably trying to find out how well-rounded and comfortable around others we were. I found out later that Stanley was a good judge of character and was good at a great many things as well. We ended up calling him Super Chief.

That second time back at St. Francis it was clear that it was the place for me. I had thought that I wanted someplace busier, like Bay State. I came to see, though, that St. Francis had the people and that made the difference. They went from last to first on my list, followed by Bay State, with my university in third. Then it was time to wait for Match Day.

Match Day is always stressful for the graduating med student and for good reason. It really can determine much of your future career. I could have saved myself a little perspiration if I had been willing to. My ten-year-old son, Tim, was a computer prodigy. He came to me about a week before the big day and asked me if I wanted to know the results of the match. He had hacked into the Match Day database and had the results all stacked neatly in his hands. Since I didn't think beginning my career with an ethical breach was such a hot idea I politely declined his offer. (Tim had also come to me at one point with a large stack of other data he had "borrowed." They were all the interior phone numbers at an intimidating federal agency as well as the phone numbers and daily access codes for Air Force One. If I had timed it right, I could have had a chat with the president. I had a chat with Tim instead.)

I did get St. Francis. So Nancy and I loaded up the van and headed out to Hartford. I found out later that I was among the top five at the university and they had taken five residents. My friends were very surprised that I hadn't matched. So I could have stayed at home after all. Looking back, though, I'm very glad we made the move. It was good for all of us to go somewhere new, we loved Connecticut, and St. Francis was even more than I hoped it would be.

Chapter 5

Trail of Blood

In Which I Try to Get Comfortable with Constant Terror

The first morning of my residency will be with me forever. On my way to St. Francis at 6:45 I felt like I was edging up to the end of a high diving board and trying to remember if I could swim. An orange Pinto pulled up next to me at a light and, for one of those irrational seconds where our feelings outrun our heads, I thought it was my med school friend, Mike. Then I remembered that he was on the other side of the continent in Washington beginning his own residency. My feeling of isolation increased.

Once I got to the OB floor it wasn't hard to find morning report; I just followed a trail of blood that went from the delivery room into the conference room. I was thinking, "Oh my God, what's that all about?" when I opened the door and there were twelve strangers sitting around a huge table: the program director, John Gibbons, assistant director, Vic Fortin, and a bunch of residents. Some of them I knew slightly from my visits and some

I didn't recognize. It's hard for someone my size to slip quietly into a meeting, but I tried.

The blood trail had been left by one of the residents who got to the meeting right before I did. He had just done a C-section with an emergency hysterectomy. His scrubs were sweat-stained, bloody, and he was still fired up from the dangerous, difficult procedure. As I was slipping into my chair he was telling the whole room what a great case it had been, all that had been demanded of his skills, and what a close call it was for the new mother. I sat there listening to all the techniques he was forced to use while comparing my skills to his. It wasn't reassuring. I thought, "I'm in the wrong place. I just haven't had enough training to do this and I'm going to kill somebody."

Then Vic Fortin, the oldest doc in the room, spoke up from his seat next to the director. "Roger, you're calling that a great case and it was *not* a great case. I'll tell what a great case is. A great case is a normal vaginal delivery with no complications."

There were a few smiles at that, and the resident dialed down his bravado. Without realizing it, I had just heard my first reading from the gospel of Vic, and I soon became a convert. Fortin always saw a case through the eyes of the patient. Whatever the medical interest or learning possibilities a case might have, the most important thing to him was that the patient had a quick, reassuring outcome. It was all about the patient and what the doctor took away from the case was secondary. That is, unfortunately, not always what you will find. There are those doctors who I have mentioned who think first of their convenience or bank account. Then there are those, like Roger, who see their work primarily as public testament to their great skills whatever the cost in worry or inconvenience to the patient. I became determined to be a Vic and not a Roger, and as I worked my way through the years from intern to chief, Vic Fortin became deeply influential to me.

As John and Vic outlined the residency schedule, though, it became clear that my path to becoming any sort of doctor at all was going to wind through the rotations far more than I had expected or wanted it to. Six months of our first year was going to be spent off-service. That meant doing things other than ob-gyn — internal medicine, newborn intensive care, and surgical intensive care. It's important to remember that a residency is yet another step in the education of a doctor, and there is still a strong emphasis on getting a well-rounded experience outside of your comfort zone. Besides the objective of rounding out the new intern's experience, the residency assignments were set up so that the least experienced residents were working with the most experienced. Each year's interns worked with the third-year residents, while the second-year residents paired up with each other. The chiefs were on call at home for all the residents.

So I was assigned to internal medicine for my first month. Great. I had just met my new colleagues and now I would be wandering in the wilderness without them. And when you're an off-service person, I soon found out, you are indeed in the wilderness — you're the outsider that gets the dregs of the cases. The interns from the particular service got the most interesting and useful cases while the off-service people got the simplest ones like asthma or non-critical diabetes. The internal medicine assignment proved to be a long and particularly trying month. Here I encountered my first ethical dilemma before I even got to my own service.

I hadn't cared for internal medicine in med school and I felt the same at St. Francis, but I did have a fine chief to work with, Mary O'Brian. This was still a time when women were well in the minority as physicians and I think that the cliché about women having to be twice as good as men to get to the same place professionally was roughly true. Mary knew her stuff cold, carried herself with quiet authority, and was greatly respected by the St. Francis staff. That wasn't always true with the patients, though, and on that first rotation there was a Jamaican man, Oliver, who couldn't get his mind around the idea of a woman doctor.

Oliver had come to the hospital with a blackened, necrotic toe. When I met him that first morning of medicine rounds I liked him. He was a friendly, charming man. But he drove Mary crazy.

"Doctor," he asked, looking at me, "What do you think the problem is?"

I, of course, deferred to the chief resident of Internal Medicine standing right next to me.

"We don't know yet, Mr. Pettijohn," Mary said, "But we will find out."

"Thank you, Nurse!"

Mary smiled at him and said, "Actually, I'm a doctor, and Dr. Kington is assisting me on your case."

He nodded and then turned and asked the rest of his questions to me. The next day it was the same thing. "Hello, Doctor! Hello, Nurse!"

That second day, Mary was a little more assertive. "Mr. Pettijohn, I am a doctor. I'm the chief resident in Internal Medicine and I'm Dr. Kington's boss."

"Ah!" And two minutes later she was "Nurse" again. It was clearly annoying her, and it was excruciating for me. I felt like an arrogant male by default and I wanted to make it clear to Mary how I felt. But first-week interns don't engage their chiefs in heart-to-hearts without being invited so I was stuck.

Eventually, she gave up. Her concern for the patient was greater than her ego and she wasn't going to badger him for respect that he clearly didn't have. I wonder how many of the male chiefs would have done the same. When we came in to see Oliver, Mary played nurse to my doctor.

"We hear you had some more pain last night. Tell Nurse and Dr. Kington all about it." It was uncomfortable, funny, and impressive.

Poor Oliver got sicker and sicker, though. The necrotic toe had been amputated in the first few days, but the source of the necrosis — which we couldn't find — kept poisoning him. His organs began to fail, and we couldn't figure out why. Diabetes is a likely culprit for necrotic tissue, but Oliver wasn't diabetic. An infection or gangrene was a possibility, but his cultures came back negative. A little over a month after his admission he was dead. I was not used to losing patients and I had liked Oliver, so I took it hard. Mary had rotated out of the unit by that time, we had a new chief, and the person who knew the case best was Oliver's attending physician. I cornered him in a conference room the day after Oliver died.

"Dr. Davis, I think we need to contact Oliver Pettijohn's family to get permission for an autopsy."

He didn't even look up at me.

"Why would we want to do an autopsy?"

"Why? My God, we need to find out if we missed something."

"That," said Davis, "Is exactly why we *don't* want to do an autopsy."

I was floored.

"Dr. Davis, if an autopsy was ever necessary this would be the case. We watched that guy waste away under our care and we need to know why."

"I don't think it's your role, Dr. Kington, to tell the attending physician what is necessary. Look," he said, "The relatives haven't asked for an autopsy. Let's not cause ourselves difficulty if we don't need to." And he walked out of the room.

He was right about the family not requesting an autopsy. Few families do. They don't like the idea of their loved one being dissected, and they don't want to surrender their time of mourning to the schedules of strangers. The new chief wasn't any more sympathetic. I happened to catch him as he was signing the death certificate. He looked a little panicked when I asked questions and rushed off.

That was my first exposure to such shameless ass-covering and it made me sick. The attending was our supervisor, too. The residents, interns, especially, were supposed to be learning from him. I guess I did learn something, but it wasn't what I expected. I certainly hadn't made it into my thirties as an innocent. I had worked in a big corporation and been through medical school, so I knew what devious self-preservation looked like. This was different. This was about the life of one patient and the lives of patients to come. It was a hell of a way to start a residency and I haven't forgotten those feelings three decades later. The one good thing about this episode was that it came at the end of that first month of medicine rotation and I was able to escape back to Ob-Gyn, a place I felt at home.

Stanley Petoski, the doc we called Super Chief, was the perfect antidote to that poisonous (in every sense) experience. He cut no corners and didn't tolerate those who did. Stanley was a tall, skinny, bespectacled, fast-talking, Polish guy from New Jersey. I don't remember which exit, but that's what he would ask about anyone who told him they were from "Joisey." Stanley was one of the smartest doctors I ever met and probably the hardest worker. He could work as hard as three doctors put together and that, strangely enough, had been empirically tested. There had been a period in which the other two residents Stanley was on rotation with were injured. One had torn his Achilles tendon and the other had injured her neck and was barely mobile in a big neck brace. Stanley covered for both of them for a month. I can tell you that a three-person rotation is exhausting, and he was on call every day for a month. I can't imagine that. Around the fifth week or so Stanley saw the resident with the neck injury out shopping without her brace. She was back on rotation the next day and Stanley had earned his nickname.

Stanley was super for other reasons as well. Some chiefs take a sink-or-swim attitude toward their interns. Watching interns sink takes less time and energy than teaching them to swim. Stanley was always there when you needed advice or guidance. He loved to teach and if you were a hard worker he loved you. He didn't abide slackers or bullshitters. Our year of residents was a good one, though, so he loved us and we loved him back.

My good friend Tony Ness was one of those residents. He was the guy that Stanley had asked about the New York Knicks in his initial interview. We had our interviews on the same weekend and I had not been impressed by Tony at all. When I saw him in the conference room on that first morning I had real questions about the standards at St. Francis. During that weekend of interviews, Tony had seemed distant, unfocused, and unresponsive to the point of rudeness. It turned out that he was just very sick. He had gotten food poisoning the day before the interview and was still not over it. As our year progressed he turned out to be very focused and very much present — a great resident and friend. That he was able to complete his interview successfully while suffering from food poisoning says a lot about his strength and dedication. Tony told me later that he hadn't been impressed with me at first, either. I always thought that it was just in return for mentioning my first impression of him. I hoped so, anyway. I didn't have an excuse.

Tony's first rotation was labor and delivery, which was lucky, but the luck stopped there. He had some very difficult cases in his first month and got the nickname Hema, because of all the blood he was using. He had a couple of major hemorrhages and, through no fault of his own, was single-handedly draining the blood bank. It took a while for that name to fade into obscurity. It's obvious that we liked nicknames. The three new residents in my year were all males and were Large, Medium, and Small. I was Large. Tony was Medium, and Craig Huttler was Small.

Then there was Vallenann. Vallenann was actually two residents, Valerie Dowling and Anna Rizzo. Both were petite blondes and were constantly being mistaken for one another, which said more about the older attendings than it said about Vallenann. A more significant similarity was that they were both very good — smart, efficient, and hard-working. Val was one of the third-year residents during my internship and she couldn't have been a better teacher, or a kinder one. I was on call on July 4th during that first year, and I was struggling.

Independence Day is probably the worst holiday to be on call for both obstetrics and the ER. For too many patients it combines long, hot days in the sun without enough hydration, lots of alcohol, and traffic jams. Add a pinch of gunpowder and stir until dangerous. So a lot of the patients I saw that day were dehydrated; some were drunk. They all thought they were in labor when, in many cases, it was the dehydration. So I got people drinking water, treated some sunburns, and the deliveries I did have were normal. But the patients were probably in better shape by the day's end than I was. I was exhausted, and inexperience and fatigue are a bad combination.

I got a phone call about 10:00 at night from a nurse on the floor who wanted to know if she could give her patient Tylenol. A simple enough question, right? Then the second guessing began. I thought it was okay. Sure. Wait, though. What if she's allergic to it? I thought back to what my pharmacology courses had told me about Tylenol. Oh, she'll be fine. But what if the Tylenol ends up masking a serious condition? Maybe the pain is telling us something.

So I called up Val. I told her that a patient had had a baby at 10:00 that morning, had a headache, and wanted some Tylenol. Would it be okay to give her some? There was a long pause on the line.

"Kevin," she said finally, "If you're going to call me every time a patient wants Tylenol we're both going to have a very long night. What do you think? Should you give the patient Tylenol?"

"Yes," I said. "Yes, I think I should."

"Then give her some," she said. "And promise not to call me again about Tylenol, okay?"

"Okay."

There are senior residents who would have ripped the heart out of an intern who did that, or who would have made a point of mentioning it later at the most embarrassing opportunity possible. I never heard a further word about it from Val.

If that had been the only time I called her needlessly and she responded beautifully, Val would still belong in my Resident's Hall of Fame. I'm ashamed to say that it was not the only time.

At another point early in my internship I got a notion in my head about a patient and wanted some advice. I don't even remember what it was about, which is a good indication of its importance. I paged Val's number and she didn't call back. That was unusual. She always called back, and it never had taken long. So I thought I might have misdialed. I paged her again and waited. Ten minutes later she hadn't called. Now that was very strange. I tried again and in a minute the conference room door burst open and Val raced in.

"Kevin! What's wrong? What happened?"

"Oh, nothing," I said happily, "I just had a question for you."

She fell into a chair, took a deep breath, and said, "If you just had a question then *why* did you page me three times in fifteen minutes?"

I really didn't have a satisfactory answer for her question. Thirty years later, though, that scene swims back into my memory when I'm getting impatient with a young doctor. Then I take a deep breath and pretend I'm Val Dowling.

The other third-year I relied upon repeatedly was Anna Rizzo, the other half of Vallenann. Anna was at the center of what is probably the most disgusting yet admirable incident in my career. It's not often that those adjectives are linked, but it was that sort of situation. To tell the story I need to note that in those days patients were prepared for labor with shaving and an enema. The shaving was to provide a more sanitary surface and the enema avoided bowel movements during the birthing process. They were both rather unnecessary and are no longer done, but during my residency they were standard procedure.

On one of my on-call nights we got a patient in labor and there was something wrong with her baby's heart rate. A normal heart rate for a full-term baby is 120 to 160 beats per minute, and this rate was dropping into the 70s every time the mother contracted. The numbers would jump back into the normal range, then drop again with the next contraction.

It was a bad situation, so we called Anna and when she did a cervical exam she found that the patient's vagina was filled with umbilical cord. The cord had come down before the baby and during every contraction it was getting squeezed and the baby's blood supply was cut. It's called a prolapsed cord and it's dangerous. It means that the doctor must insert her hand into the vagina and hold the baby's head up and away from the umbilical cord until a C-section can be done.

Anna had been "brought up right," as we say of a well-trained doctor, so she immediately jumped onto the patient's bed, got down under the sheets and inserted her hand to hold up the baby's head. We rushed the bed down a crowded hall to the C-section room and started to work. By now Anna was on the floor, hidden in bed sheets and surgical drapes, her right arm up in the air holding the baby's head. Then the anesthesia hit the patient and the enema released. It sounded like a small explosion and we heard Anna scream as feces rolled down her arm and under her uniform. We tried to keep working as fast as we could while she called out the baby's pulse in a muffled voice and pleaded "Please hurry." But someone had started laughing and once the rest of us started, progress began to slow.

We finally got to the baby. I found the head, tapped Anna's hand to let her know that she could release, and then made the delivery. It took eight or nine minutes from the emergency call to a healthy baby. That's not bad, especially considering the laughter, but God knows how long it seemed to Anna down in her dark, hot, stinking, claustrophobic little hell. She crawled out slowly from beneath the drapes and kind of wobbled off without saying a word. When we cleaned up and went to find her she was in the call room taking a shower. She was in there for ninety minutes. It was the longest shower anyone had ever taken in the call room and every second of it was deserved. Anna is also in my Residents Hall of Fame with a special commendation for conspicuous dedication. And then some.

The third third-year resident was T.D., and he was a different sort of person entirely: arrogant, critical, stubborn, and thoroughly unpleasant. The residents laughed about the days that T.D. seemed to be "off his meds" and at his worst. It wasn't as simple as moods though. His behavior was fine with patients and even sycophantic with superiors. Perhaps there was some sort of resentment working on T.D., but I never cared enough to try to find out. T.D. was a strong believer in the old school of intern hazing. I don't respond well to bullying, though, and early on we had a run-in that defined the rest of our relationship.

I was on call in the ER one morning about 2:00 and saw a patient that I thought had a ruptured ectopic pregnancy. She was in a great deal of pain. So I paged T.D. and told him that he needed to come down to the OR because we had to operate on this woman immediately. For that I needed the supervision of a senior resident.

"Oh no, you're not!" he yelled when I mentioned operating. "You're not operating on anybody until I see them."

"I understand that," I said, "Can you come in and take a look though?"

"I don't think I even need to come in, judging by your story. It doesn't sound like an ectopic to me."

This was just mean-spirited stonewalling and I told him that if he didn't come in I was going to take her to the OR myself. I couldn't really do that, but had I tried, it would have created enough of a mess for T.D. that the threat carried a bit of weight. So he reluctantly and angrily got out of bed and came down to the hospital.

We were in the ER and he was examining the patient when he said, "I don't think she has an ectopic pregnancy. We're going to have to do a culdocentesis."

A culdocentesis was an old-school test that we did before we got ultrasound. You'd do a pelvic exam and insert a needle into the abdominal cavity to see if there was any blood in there. This was during the infancy of ultrasound, so it wasn't unheard of that he wanted to do the test, but it was unusual and, in this case, unnecessary. This woman had an ectopic pregnancy; I'm sure he knew it, and he just wanted to delay admitting that I was right. It wouldn't be hard to find out, though. If my diagnosis was right there would most definitely be blood in there, and probably a lot of it.

"Okay, T.D.," I said, and got the patient set up on the examination table.

I inserted a speculum and I could see an ominous, blue, bulging mass. It sure looked like blood to me and it sure looked like it was under a lot of pressure. T.D. looked himself, then looked at me and said, "That's just a normal cul-de-sac."

He took the needle, stuck it in, and a jet of blood shot out, smacked him in the face, and hit the wall behind him. He turned to look at me with a scowl on his face, dripping with blood, and it was like a cue in a stage comedy.

"So T.D.," I asked, "is that a *positive* culdocentesis or a *negative*?"

We took her to the OR. Not being able to keep my mouth shut might have ruined my relationship with T.D., but since it was terrible anyway, that was pretty much beside the point.

So those were the fellow residents who introduced me to St. Francis and my residency. With one exception, I couldn't have asked for a better bunch to go through boot camp with. And even T.D. had his educational value. The cast kept changing, of course. Chiefs left the hospital, third-years took their places, and we all advanced. That first cast of characters, though, was formative for me, and at their head were Gibbons and Fortin. From the first day in the conference room it was clear that they were completely different sorts of doctors, but they were both excellent and they complemented one another.

John Gibbons had been sitting at the head of that big table on my first morning. Gibbons was proper in manner and speech, and careful in his dress — an Ivy Leaguer who was something of a snob. He had been trained in New York City hospitals as a surgeon and then became an obstetrician. Highly skilled and urbane, he could be quite witty, but his formality kept him at arm's length socially. One of the chief residents called him by his first name one day during surgery.

"Many of my colleagues, Doctor," Gibbons answered, "are on a first-name basis with me, but none of the residents are."

Another young resident once told a group of us that she needed "to go pee." Gibbons made it very clear to her that such language was unacceptable for a physician.

Gibbons might sound unpleasant, but he wasn't. His style would never be mine, but I learned a lot from him about self-respect and standards of behavior in the medical profession. He did things to try to help the residents with their cultural betterment. He took us to fine restaurants occasionally and once had members of the Hartford Opera come to the hospital. They explained opera to us and sang parts of a few arias. I always liked him for trying to broaden our horizons. Gibbons could be patronizing and endearing at the same time. His tendency toward snobbery could be funny, though. One day he was meeting a new group of residents and one of them had a very impressive name: Remington Brooks III. Gibbons thought he had found an Ivy League compatriot.

"You sound as if you might be from Harvard, Dr. Brooks," he said.

"Naw," said Brooks, "Utah."

Unflappable, Gibbons just turned to one of the other new people, a woman named Casey Kelly.

"Well, Dr. Kelly, what a fine Irish name. Are you from Notre Dame?"

"No," Casey said, "Yale."

The whole room burst out laughing. We were all well aware of Gibbons's snobbish tendencies, but it was affectionate laughter nonetheless.

Gibbons had a reputation as a gifted technician in the OR and I saw that for myself one day in a memorable way. We had a private patient who had had a Caesarean hysterectomy. That's a very bloody process, and she had continued to bleed. Her attending was a devout Muslim and was unavailable on this particular holy day because he was praying. The bleeding was becoming dangerous and since we couldn't reach her physician, we called John Gibbons.

"Get her to the OR, and I'll come in myself," he said.

We got the woman prepped, and she was the sickest patient I had ever seen. She was bleeding out and it was frightening. There were three anesthesiologists where there is normally one, and two of them were squeezing blood bags trying to get it into the patient as fast as they could. They kept telling us to hurry, which was hardly necessary, but it showed the dire situation we were in.

Gibbons walked in quietly, started to work, and dissected through the bloody mess in front of him with the calmest, quickest, smoothest surgery I'd ever seen. He never hesitated out of uncertainty or paused to think about what to do next. It was like watching a confident artist sketching. This was a very tricky procedure, too. You have to go deep down into the pelvic area and tie off the hypogastrics. The hypogastric artery and vein are right next to each other. You have to get a clamp around the artery without pinching the vein, which has a very thin wall. If you tear the vein it's almost impossible to repair and your patient is in big trouble.

All you have to do, then, is reach down into a blood-filled pelvic cavity, feel around for an artery and vein that you can barely see and which are dangerously close to one another, separate them, and clamp the right one without damaging the other. Then you need to put in sutures. Gibbons reached in and I thought he must still be feeling around for the artery when one of the anesthesiologists said, "What did you do? She's looking stable for the first time."

Gibbons had already clamped the artery. In another minute he had gotten sutures in there and the patient's vital signs were nearing normal. I had never seen anything like it. Admittedly, I didn't have much experience at that point, but I do now, and what he was able to do that night still amazes me.

So the patient was stabilized and eventually her attending showed up, thanked Gibbons at length, and asked him a favor. "John, I'm flying back to Pakistan tonight and I'll be gone for a week, so I'd appreciate it if you'd take care of this patient for me."

Gibbons, in his urbane Upper East Side accent said, "Malick, don't worry about a thing. I'll take care of everything."

I thought, "Wow. Here's the busy chair, director of our program, it's the middle of the night, and he's going to take care of this patient he just met. What a guy. That's why he is where he is."

As soon as Malick left, Gibbons turned to me and said, "Dr. Kington, you're going to check on this patient every twenty minutes for the rest of the night. If there are any problems call the chief resident." Then he went home.

That smooth and instinctual sense of hospital politics was as much a part of John Gibbons as his phenomenal skills. *All* of that was why he was where he was.

Vic Fortin, on the other hand, was not subtle or political. He was a big bear of a guy who had been in private practice for years after he quit playing football for the Green Bay Packers. He had seen everything and had done, according to him, a hundred thousand deliveries. Vic was a salt-of-the-earth general ob-gyn who was very practical. If you needed specific guidance on a procedure, he was the guy you asked. I never once heard him quote an article. Instead, he always talked about patients he had seen and things that he had done.

Vic was also one of the early adopters of ultrasound. It fit his practical approach perfectly and he became, late in his career, an amazing ultrasonographer when very few others were doing it. He gave us a detailed diagnosis through his ultrasounds that we couldn't believe was possible. You can't tell what cell type a tumor is by doing that, but he managed somehow.

"Kevin, I've got a mucinous cystadenocarcinoma of the ovary here."

"Dr. Fortin, you did a biopsy?"

"No, I don't need a biopsy. I'm just telling you what it is."

Shades of Big Ed Fields. He was as good as Big Ed at diagnosis as well. We residents tried for four years to catch him in a wrong diagnosis and we never did.

Patients loved Vic. I had never seen the sort of trust and affection for a doctor that Vic's patients had for him. It was striking. I remember the two of us entering the room of a woman who had recently given birth and who was weakening, complaining of abdominal pain, and very frightened. Vic had delivered one of her older children and when she saw him walk into the room her relief was visible. He chatted with her casually, brought in an ultrasound unit, did a reading and discovered some hemorrhaging. She needed to have immediate surgery and that can scare a patient badly. With Vic it was different.

"Maggie, you've got a little bit of bleeding in there and we're going to get you up to the OR and fix that. That's okay with you, isn't it?"

"Sure, Dr. Fortin."

Nurses loved him, too. He saw their difficult work through their eyes and never made it harder than it needed to be. Walking down the floor with him was always fun.

"Ellen," he said to a nurse who had done him a favor, "Why is someone like you working in a place like this?"

"Tina, if I were only thirty years younger I'd take you out of this hellhole."

Corny stuff, but there was a real person there and that's what the nurses and the patients responded to. Vic liked people and he cared about people and that's what came across. Both John Gibbons and Vic Fortin were models for me. I very much hoped that I would one day be as adept and confident an operator as John and have some portion of the practical genius and human touch that Vic had. The truth is that, whatever our ambitions, we all reflect the glints of our influences through our own character and tendencies. At that point in my first year, though, I was just trying to keep my head above water. I was unsure of myself, almost always worried, and felt that I was usually only one step ahead of disaster. I was, in other words, an intern.

Chapter 6

Teachers and Students

*In Which I Learn That There's No Guard Rail
on the Learning Curve*

John Gibbons. Vic Fortin. Stan Petoski. Val Dowling. Anna Rizzo. I was very lucky to begin an internship with such teachers. And even here at the threshold of my medical career I was beginning to recognize the deep relationship between the practice of medicine and the teaching of it. The things that make people good doctors are the same things that make them good teachers — a gift for observation, empathy, and cooperation. All of these people saw what each younger resident needed for motivation and reassurance, and they were willing to provide it. They ignored the green, self-doubting neophyte you were and respected the doctor that they thought you could become. Why? That's a question that I've asked myself many times as teaching has become more and more what I do myself. What makes a good teacher? These were great people, but they weren't saints. There was ego to be found there and competitiveness. But there

was also a commitment to medicine beyond one's own career —
an ability to see the big picture professionally and that makes all
the difference.

Those morning conferences were a seminar in John
Gibbons's style of teaching. As we gathered around the big table
he went through the case reports and new admissions, asking the
residents to describe and evaluate each patient. "Putting your oar
in the water," as John always expressed it. He typically started
with interns, let them get to the point where they'd start to fumble
or hesitate, then draw in a second-year to assist. The second-
years added what they knew and maybe threw in some
references from the literature. Then the third-years were asked if
we had covered everything. The third-years were glad to top off
the discussion if they could. John made them feel like the experts
in the room while actually testing them. He was a very smart man.
The whole process was collegial, cooperative, and highly
effective. I suppose the shark-tank approach that some residents
face could be effective in its own intimidating way, but I'm sure
that in those programs a lot of energy spent on ass-covering and
excuse-making is diverted from learning.

There were some good teachers outside of ob-gyn, too, and
since much of the intern's year was spent on other rotations that
was important. A few of the outside residents looked at OBs as
accessories at best. They gave you the simple cases — the
asthmatic or the GI bleeder. If you were lucky and they had a
pregnant woman with a medical problem then they might say,

"Give it to the OB intern." On rounds, though, or in question sessions, they really didn't spend much time with you. They saw themselves as there to teach their own interns and we were just allowed to ride along.

Bud Ardellino, on the other hand, my favorite internal medicine attending, treated me like one of his own people and went out of his way to make the material relevant to me. If we saw a patient with hypothyroidism he'd ask, "What if this patient were pregnant and had this condition? What would change in your management?" The same thing was true if a patient had hypertension.

"Kevin, tell everybody how much different hypertension is for your specialty."

It is indeed very different in a pregnant woman and can be a sign of a serious condition called toxemia. Then it's not just run-of-the-mill high blood pressure you're treating. The disease includes hypertension but is far more complex and dangerous. The same caution has to be taken with diabetes. An OB will control sugar levels far more strictly in a pregnant woman because the life of the mother and the baby can be endangered. The way Bud brought out that information from the OB interns helped them and it helped his internal medicine people. It was the big-picture approach again, and Bud was great at it.

It felt good to be able to answer questions about my specialty to other doctors. I knew the material. Most competent interns do. It's the practical problem of applying that knowledge to a particular patient in a stressful situation that the intern lacks. Vic Fortin, of course, was always the guy to go to for the practical side of things. In morning conference, after John was done with his fatherly grilling, Vic jumped in with something memorable from his very long experience.

"Just remember, guys, that you're not dealing with medical conditions here, you're dealing with people who have medical conditions."

"Let's say you run across an STD (i.e., a sexually transmitted disease) in a patient you've tested for pregnancy. Don't go blundering into the exam room with that in your head before you think over how to say it. And you'd better check to see if she's got a husband the size of the White Refrigerator waiting outside. You'd better *really* think that over!"

The White Refrigerator was me. In the middle 80s there was a very famous, very large, football player for the Chicago Bears named William "Refrigerator" Perry, and Vic liked describing me as the Caucasian version of The Fridge.

Vic Fortin got more laughs in ten minutes than John Gibbons did in a year, yet there was practical wisdom in what he said that I'm still using thirty years later. But, however well you know the material and however good the practical advice you've been given, there's no substitute for the peculiarities of life on a hospital floor — and they can be very peculiar indeed. I had to learn to rely on myself, and the learning curve was steep.

Within the first few weeks of my intern year it looked like I might get dangerously on the wrong side of one of our chiefs, Julie Henderson. In the short time I had known her, Dr. Henderson struck me as an unusual person — very intense and earnest. Part of that strangeness derived from the fact that she was a repeater. When you were presenting a patient to her she repeated what you just told her as if she was the one telling it to you. It was disconcerting. This night she was going off duty and caught me by the arm in the hall.

"Kevin, you've got to take care of a patient I just saw in clinic! She's a mess. She's got breast cancer, ovarian cancer, and maybe uterine cancer. She's got a really big uterus, a big ovarian mass, a breast lump. We need to work her up right now. She needs a biopsy of that breast and probably a hysterectomy, oncology staging ..." On and on. Julie was amped.

She wanted me to do the pre-op H and P, so I went into the patient's room, talked to her, and she was cordial, relaxed, and didn't seem to have any complaints. She had simply come into the clinic for an annual Pap smear. I was beginning to feel confused, so I started my exam and my confusion increased. I couldn't find a breast mass; her uterus seemed a normal size; I couldn't feel the ovarian mass. It was alarming. I thought that my examination skills must be so bad that I was missing everything. I came out of the room very disheartened and wandered down to the nurses' station to write up the H and P. I guess I looked like a lonely orphan, because Super Chief walked by and said, "Kevin, you look miserable. What's wrong?"

I said, "Stan, I really have doubts about my exam skills. Julie gave me a cancer patient to do an H and P on and I can't find anything wrong. I'm missing everything!"

Stan said, "Where is she? What's her room number? Let me go check her."

We went into the room together, Stanley talked to her for a while, examined her, and then we went back out to the hall.

"Discharge that patient, Kevin!" he said. "There's not a thing wrong with her."

Oh, my God, I thought, I've got one chief telling me to work her up and do all sorts of critical stuff and another one telling me to discharge her.

I said, "Stan, I can't do that. Julie wanted me to admit her and run a lot of tests."

"She'll be okay it," he said. "Send this woman home. She's fine."

Well, I thought, this is it for me. I'm going to discharge this patient and tomorrow morning Julie's going to come in, find out, and blow a gasket. All night I was turning it over in my mind as I went from one case to another, occasionally trying to grab some food or a few minutes of rest. Morning report rushed around at 7:00, though, and it was time to mount the gallows.

The conference room was full; Julie was sitting next to John Gibbons and he was shuffling through the night's admission forms.

"Julie," he said, "I see that you admitted a patient from the clinic."

"Yes," she said, "Kevin took the H and P and did the exam. What did you find, Kevin?"

This was it. "Well, I examined her," I said and hesitated. "And I thought that she was all right. So I sent her home."

Julie had to be completely flabbergasted. After everything she had told me, how could she not be? But, of course, all she said was, "She was all right. He sent her home."

After all that tension all night long I almost laughed out loud. Almost.

So I began to look at myself and my own judgment in a different way. Maybe I was capable of a solid diagnosis even if a senior doctor disagreed with me. At the same time, I was learning to see the patient in a new way. It's too easy to let the power of being a doctor blind you to the individualities, the unique qualities, of every patient. As Vic would say these were not medical conditions but people who had them. There was a patient that first year who showed me how clever, creative, and independent patients can be.

I inherited Duffy my first day on the internal medicine service. Duffy was known to all the medical interns because he'd been in the hospital for ten months. Duffy was a very sick man.

He had cancer, diabetes, congestive heart failure, kidney disease. Everyone knew that he was dying. The intern who turned him over to me was very happy, because it meant that now if Duffy died he wouldn't have to do his dictation. A dictation involves looking up and recording everything on record about a patient since admission — all the tests, labs, x-rays, scans, reports, diagnoses. You have to tell the patient's whole story from admission until death and after eleven months that can be a long story.

One of the internal medicine interns made himself famous by doing a dictation on a patient who had been in the hospital for about as long as Duffy. It consisted of something like "John Smith was admitted on November 2, 1986, for chest pain and had multiple other medical problems. He got sicker and sicker and sicker and finally he died." His brilliant attempt was shot down by medical records, unfortunately, so the intern had to do the whole history, but he won the admiration of everyone who had been forced to do a long dictation.

Duffy was a resourceful man. Every night he somehow removed his feeding tube. The tube went down his nose and it's very uncomfortable so it's understandable that he'd want it out. How he managed to get it out himself isn't nearly as understandable. If you were the intern on Duffy's service you had to put in a feeding tube every night for, whatever its inconvenience, it was keeping him alive. I spent the whole month of my Medicine rotation trying to figure out how to keep him from taking out that damned tube. By the end of the month he was restrained in four-point restraints; he was in a straitjacket so that he could sit up in his chair and sleep. I put his feeding tube in and taped it to his neck with a lot of tape. Then about 2:00 in the morning the phone rang.

"Dr. Kington? Duffy needs to have his feeding tube replaced."

So I hauled myself down there to find Duffy sitting there in his wheelchair, in the straitjacket, in the four-point restraints, and he was laughing a soft little laugh.

I said, "Duffy, damn it, how did you get that feeding tube out?"

"Heh, heh, heh, heh, heh …"

I never figured it out. This was a guy who could barely move. I asked his nurses to watch him carefully, but they never could catch him doing it.

Another of those early patients on the Medicine service was an old woman who told me that she was going to die that night. She said it with fear and sadness that touched me, but also with a certainty that was chilling. I had been called to see her because she had a gastric ulcer and some gastrointestinal bleeding. It was concerning but didn't seem life-threatening. She was sure she was dying, though, because she had coughed a small amount blood. I told her that that wasn't uncommon with an ulcer and set up a soothing wash to reduce the bleeding.

Then she looked up at me and said, "I really feel terrible." And she stopped breathing. Her vitals were gone, and we couldn't resuscitate her. She was dead.

Many patients fear that they're dying, of course, and say so. There was something in the way she said it, though, that has stayed with me all this time. Another of Vic's mottos is "Listen to the patient."

That case was notable, too, because I almost got myself in trouble. When I came on duty I discovered that the intern on the previous shift had ignored this patient despite her complaints and the bleeding. I had been, after twelve hours, the first doctor to see her. That intern came sidling into the room right after the woman had been declared and I was angry. We had done all that we could do for the patient physically, but she had lain in that bed for a long time frightened and in need of a doctor's reassurance. When only the two of us were in the room I grabbed the intern by the front of his scrubs and pushed him into the wall and screamed at him. I like to think that it happened because I was very tired and had just lost a patient, but there was no excuse for what I did. I must say, though, that it gave me a lot of satisfaction to see blood drops from the patient flying off me onto his glasses and to see the look of fear behind those lenses. There were, fortunately, no repercussions for me, but then that's not the sort of thing that the intern would have wanted to bring attention to. I did get a thank-you note for tearing into the intern from one of the nurses.

Bev Tanner was another patient who gave me a lesson on listening. She called me from her home one night when I was on OB rotation because she thought she was going into labor. Anna Rizzo was my third-year and checked in on me later.

"Anything going on tonight?"

"Well," I said, "I just told a patient to come in who sounds like she's in labor."

"Was it Bev Tanner?"

"Yeah, why?" I said, and she started laughing.

"You'll find out."

"Come on," I said, "tell me."

"Well, Bev Tanner calls every night. She gets worried. You probably could have told her to stay home until she was a little further along, because she's never in labor."

Twenty minutes later Bev arrived, and she was delivering her baby. She probably had been in fifteen times in the last two weeks and finally she was right. So even when the patient isn't right the first (or fourteenth) time, don't stop listening.

And then in the course of an intern's education there are simply the nights when all hell breaks loose. One can never underestimate the teaching value of chaos. A patient came in whose husband was a fundamentalist preacher. She had labor, delivered her baby, then went into seizures. Any OB would know what was happening to her; this was preeclampsia turning into eclampsia. But the husband thought he knew what was happening, too — that his wife had been possessed by the devil, and he was determined to do something about it.

We called a code, started hanging magnesium drips, and ordered Valium to break the seizure. While all that was going on, the husband lay down on the floor next to the examination table and started speaking in tongues. He was on his back doing a sort of bacon-in-the-skillet thing — rolling from his shoulders to his hips, waving his arms and riffing like a demented auctioneer.

We were stepping over him trying to get the drips going. It was tricky because there were a lot of tubes and cords getting moved around and the flailing tended to get in the way. For a few insane minutes we had a patient in full seizure on the exam table, her husband in seizure on the floor, and resuscitation procedures getting barked out over a background of high-volume gibberish. Eventually, the magnesium and Valium began to grab, and the patient stopped seizing. She was lying on the table, post-seizure and confused while her husband was still on his back, writhing around the floor and yipping. Then the code team ran in, sized up the situation, and the anesthesiologist bent down next to the preacher and started getting a pulse from his neck.

I pointed towards the patient and yelled, "Not him! Her!"

More confusion.

Pointing again, "*He's* not the one seizing. *She* is."

The preacher was just about to get intubated when things finally got under control. The patient was stable, the code team packed up and left, and eventually the husband realized that he had been successful, so he quieted down and pulled up a chair next to his wife.

I was able to handle that madness, and as the year went on I was starting to think that I might get through the internship with no major disasters. As I look back on that year one of the measuring sticks could be called the "laparoscopy scale." Laparoscopy is a surgical procedure that uses a remote, lighted surgical instrument. The incision can be very small compared to traditional surgery, and you can, of course, see what you're doing in otherwise inaccessible places. It was brand new at this time — around the mid-80s.

On my first laparoscopy as an intern I was working under a young attending two years out of her residency, and I was really excited to try the new technique. She asked me how many of these procedures I had done.

"This is my first one."

She was not impressed and said, "Well, then, I'll do this one." She inserted a needle into the belly button and blew air into the abdomen to allow for easier viewing and movement. Then she started looking. She looked and looked (in those days there wasn't a display screen, just a little eyepiece) and I was getting antsier by the minute as I watched her peering into the instrument. Finally I broke a bit of protocol by asking if I could take a look.

"No," she said, and didn't even look up

Ouch.

Later she apologized. The needle had gone where it shouldn't have, and we had to call in a vascular surgeon to correct the damage. Thank God she hadn't let me insert the needle or I would never have wanted to do another laparoscopy. Her answer, in any case, was an object lesson in where I ranked in the pecking order of the OR. By the third or fourth laparoscopy, though, I was doing everything — inserting the needle and the gas and doing as much looking as I wanted. I was building confidence, but it was still nerve-racking. There was always the danger of puncturing the anterior vena cava, as that attending had done.

During one of the laparoscopy procedures I was with an attending and a med student. I had inserted the needle and inflated the abdomen, and the attending was looking, but going very slowly and carefully. There was also a distinct smell of intestinal gas. I was worried about where the needle might have gone and so, clearly, was the attending.

"Kevin," he said, "I don't see evidence of it, but there's an intestinal smell that worries me. I think we might have punctured the bowel." Uh-oh. My stomach dropped. I had thought I was getting good at this.

Then the med student began to fidget and finally said, "Uh, Doctor that was me. I just ... uh ..."

The attending was a rather proper guy, but even he had to put down the scope for a moment to laugh. More importantly to me, I hadn't screwed up. Seeing my progress in those first-year laparoscopies was a big deal for me.

You do a lot of C-sections as an intern and D and Cs (dilation and curettage). You pretty much just watch the hysterectomies, because they can be so difficult, and, of course, when something goes wrong with whatever you're doing you get pulled out of the driver's seat in a hurry. The uncomfortable truth, though, is that you really learn more from the screw-ups and the disasters than you do from the flawless procedures. Just by watching a procedure that's gone wrong, a C-section for example, you really can improve your technique and your confidence level. It's invaluable to see first-hand that a bad situation can be retrieved if you keep your composure, rely on what you know, and rely on the team around you. That's a good antidote to self-doubt, and if you let it, self-doubt can gnaw at you as a doctor — certainly as an intern.

Self-doubt might seem an unusual characteristic for a doctor, but, with the possible exception of surgeons, it's not. Those physical and mental demands made in dangerous situations can be quite humbling. There's a mental attitude that's easy to fall into called the imposter syndrome. When you're surrounded by very competent people and you are painfully aware of what you don't know, it's easy to ignore what you do know. You can begin to feel like you're the incompetent in the bunch and only by luck and hard work have you been able to hide the fact. You feel like you're always one step away from being found out. I've talked to people in other professions who have felt the imposter syndrome, so I know it's not uncommon. That doesn't make it any less uncomfortable when you're caught in it.

The first morning conference at St. Francis I had felt like an imposter. I remembered how I felt listening to the other docs' exploits and thinking that they were simply beyond my ability. In the interim I had discovered a lot about myself, my patients, and my colleagues.

The defining story of my intern year came, appropriately enough, right at the tail end. My friend Tony Ness called one night. He was fairly busy up in labor and delivery, but I was getting no calls from the ER at all. So I tried to get a nap to counteract the chronic sleep-deprivation of that first year. I was drifting somewhere in stage one sleep when the phone rang.

"We have an emergency C-section on a private patient. There's no time to get her attending in here. I need you right now."

I said, "Okay," then I hung up the phone, sat up in bed, put my shoes on, and instantly fell back to sleep. I was that tired.

Two minutes later Tony burst into the room, shook me awake, and said, "Are you coming or not?"

I said, "Coming? What for?"

He gave me a few more shakes and in a moment we were running down the hallway to the OR and we did our stat C-section. The notable thing was that we did it all on our own without getting anyone's advice or permission. We made the decision, readied the room, assembled the team, and did it.

When it was over I got a moment to think about it and it felt good. That's when I knew that the previous year had made a difference in me. I was getting prepared for covering the house. It also felt good that after the patient was on the way back to her room one of the senior nurses turned to us and said, "Nice job." She knew what it had meant, too.

Chapter 7

Sophomore

In Which I Learn to Rely on Dr. Kington

The years of a residency change rapidly. There's no comfortable vacation between them that allows you to review and recharge. On June 30th I was an intern. On July 1st I was a second-year and suddenly everything changed. It was peculiar and wonderful. It felt as if I had returned from a long, tiring trip and was home. Now I would be on call with a peer because all three residents on the call schedule were second-years. There were no more off-service rotations; all my work would be in ob-gyn. Most importantly, I felt that I belonged there at St. Francis, not like that terrified ex-med student who followed a trail of blood into morning conference just last summer. I had spent a year in this place, and six months with my OB staff.

The intern year is when residents learn the most — certainly in part because they don't know much to begin with. It's baptism by fire and you certainly get tempered. During the second year you begin to put an edge on your skills. Because the call schedule contains just second-years, unless there's an emergency, you don't hand off procedures to senior residents. You're it. You do the most surgeries and the most deliveries you'll ever do in the residency program. You also start learning more difficult procedures, especially hysterectomies. The decision to come to St. Francis looked better than ever in that respect. If a residency program is too inbred — if there are no practitioners trained outside the program — you get lots of doctors doing the same thing the same way. It's far better to see a range of approaches. At St. Francis everybody had a little different style.

Since we worked with peers the second year, we relied primarily on our attending physicians to show us the more advanced techniques. There were the young hotshots who had just gotten out of their residencies and there were the old-timers who had been doing it their way for decades. We liked the hotshots because they let us do more than the old guys did. They were practically peers, and they trusted the residents. They also knew all the latest techniques. That period in the first half of the 80s introduced some new and very useful procedures that literally became standard operating procedure. That was the year when I first saw videos of laparoscopic surgeries done by the Nezhat brothers of Atlanta. Change was happening, and the young guys were enthusiastic about it. The old-timers, of course, were more cautious, but their ways of doing things had been tested thousands of times. I loved both groups of attendings, but I probably learned more of lasting value from the old-timers.

Ron Fishman was one of them. He'd been practicing for thirty-some years when I worked with him. Ron was one of the most careful and meticulous doctors I had ever seen or have ever seen since. His mantra was, "Is it dry?" Before closing the patient when we did a hysterectomy Ron was obsessive about making sure that the area where the uterus had been showed absolutely no sign of bleeding. None. We looked and looked, wiped the operative site, and then looked again.

"Is it dry?"

"Ron, it's dry. Let's close."

It began to drive me a little crazy. I made up analogies to get the point across.

"Ron, it reminds me of the Sahara Desert."

"Ron, when the Mojave Desert grows up it wants to be this patient."

It made him laugh, but it never reassured him and we kept on looking. What a great lesson for a young resident, though. Ron implanted in me the idea that the operative site had to be perfect. That's especially true in laparoscopies. The gas that's used to fill the abdomen and separate the organs can also provide enough pressure to stop bleeding. Then when you close and the pressure drops back to normal, the hemorrhaging starts. Ron's carefulness is something I still teach, and I've probably driven a few young doctors crazy. Their patients are better off.

There was another Ron who was an older attending — Ron Czaja. He was careful, too, and it showed in his slow, deliberate style. He could not be hurried for any reason. If a baby was crowning when he walked into the delivery room, he was the same calm doctor that he was sitting at his desk.

"Doctor Czaja, hurry. The baby is crowning."

"My God, haven't you ever seen a baby born before? They don't just fall out."

Czaja was also extremely careful about bleeding — even on the way in. There are plenty of operators who, even if they're careful about closing dry, will be pretty cavalier about staunching the small vessels as they cut through the fascia. Ron Czaja zapped every last bleeder with an electric wand called a Bovie. It took us five minutes to get through the fascia when it took less careful docs half that at most. The main thing that Ron Czaja taught me was that rushing wasn't, except in the direst emergencies, a necessity. It was an option. During my fourth year, we residents gave each other nicknames based on which attending we were supposed to resemble. They called me Ron Czaja. I was a little offended to be thought of as that slow and deliberate. It wouldn't bother me now; in the intervening years I very definitely have become like Ron Czaja.

Another of the older attendings was Ted Gutkowski. What I learned from Ted was less about technique or standards of care and more about very practical ways to approach a patient. He was a little like Vic Fortin as far as stressing the practical, but in a more negative sense. The first time I scrubbed with Ted he told me he wanted one thing.

"Dr. Kington, during this case we are going to maintain radio silence."

"I'm not sure I understand what you mean, Doctor Gutkowski."

"I mean I do not want you to speak during the case. Not one word. If you need an instrument, point to it. If you see something unusual, point to it. Do *not* mention it."

I thought he was a strange man, and then he told me his story. He had had at least a couple of young residents who caused him a whole lot of trouble with patients. One of them had helped Ted deliver a baby that had a noticeable anomaly.

The resident said loudly, "What the hell is *that*?"

The mother, of course, was conscious.

Another time a young doctor said, "Oops!" during a tough delivery. Thus was born Ted Gutkowski's radio silence requirement.

On the other side of the coin from the old guys was Kenny Gordon. Kenny G was one of the young hotshots who let the residents do a lot of the work. That was very useful because however great the lessons from the older guys, you still needed to get the reps yourself. Kenny G was always good for that. He was famous for taking young residents aside while they were scrubbing, lean into their faces, and whisper, "I only have one thing to say about this case." Pause. "Don't fuck up."

Then he backed off, laughed, and then it was all on you. It was funny, but it also let the resident know that he or she was on probation. Kenny G might give the residents a long leash, but there was a leash.

So, with Kenny G's sage advice ringing in my ears, and trying to balance the styles of the old guys with that of the young guys, I began to learn how to do the more complex surgeries — hysterectomies and tumor reductions. There's a lot to learn, and there's a reason that you wait until the second year to try. The uterus is a large organ and, of course, there's a massive blood supply that must be controlled. There are a lot of things that can go wrong and so there were restrictions on what we second-years could handle. The cancer cases went to the chiefs and the attending oncologists. Twins and triplets went upstairs as well. I was so glad to get the procedures I did, though, because the most important thing with all the gynecological procedures was the amount of hands-on time you got in the OR. Watching is useful; doing is crucial.

Hysterectomies aren't a difficult operation in themselves, but a lot depends on why the operation is necessary and the complications that can result from that. Usually you're doing the procedure because of heavy bleeding, fibroids, or pelvic pain. Depending on what causes those symptoms it can be an easy hysterectomy or a tricky one. When they're difficult you can run into a lot of adhesions or endometriosis, which is an inflammation of the uterine wall that can generate growths and cysts. The fibroids could be very large or in a very inconvenient place and that could cause problems as well.

Most of the hysterectomies that you get as a second-year are of two types: the simple parts of the difficult cases or all of the simple cases. Every hysterectomy — and C-section, for that matter — starts with an exploratory laparotomy. A second-year learns to do that over and over. Then once you've seen what you need to see you go in. (Laparoscopic hysterectomies, by the way, where you do the whole procedure through a tiny incision, hadn't come along when I was a second-year. The Nezhats were doing them in Atlanta, but not us. We did other procedures that way, though, such as tubals, taking out ovaries, and taking out cysts. The first hysterectomy I did that way was in my fourth year when I was a chief.) So in those days a normal second-year was as good as any doctor ever was at opening up an abdomen and closing it. Of course, it's always that pesky part in between that keeps you on your toes.

Here's the drill. You begin an entry by opening up the broad ligament at the round ligaments, then dissect down so that you can see the anatomy. You want a clear view of as much real estate as you can get. Next you go after the blood supply sequentially. As long as you're lucky enough to see the veins and arteries you need to get at, you just clamp, cut, tie, clamp, cut, tie over and over. Clamp the artery, cut around the clamp, and tie off. Then on to the next artery. In the best of circumstances it's very easy. The problem is those complications. The best attendings let you go on your own until you started getting over your head, then they stepped in with some close guidance or just take over themselves. The best of the best always let you get to that turning point then pushed you just a little bit further. With those teachers you learned something new every time you scrubbed with them.

As always, though, there were the docs who were the great teachers and there were those who didn't try. One memorable moment in our St. Francis teaching annals involved Remington Brooks III, the intern whose name had so impressed John Gibbons. Brooks was now a second-year along with Tony, Craig, and me, although he was in surgery. Still, he scrubbed with us occasionally on the cases where we needed one of his surgery mentors. During one procedure the attending wasn't letting him do much of anything. He worked and worked and Brooks, clearly getting antsy, asked if he could step in and do something.

"No," said the attending. "You're not ready."

"I've done some appendectomies."

"I know," said the attending. "I want to do this."

His head turned back to the table and he worked and worked some more. Finally, he looked up and said, "Dr. Brooks, tie off this artery."

Remington stepped in and tied off and that was that. We were done.

As the attending stepped away from the table he said, "Dr. Brooks, when you dictate this case be sure to mention all the details of the techniques we used." Remington Brooks III replied

"I'll tell you what, Doctor. When *you* dictate this case and you get to the part where you need a suture cut just let me know and I'll come down and dictate that for you."

Everyone was silent for a very long moment. Residents just didn't talk like that to attendings. Then the attending laughed, clapped Brooks on the shoulder, and we all began to breathe again. Remington won our admiration for sheer chutzpah. Surgeons.

I also got a lot of experience doing what I called "Catholic tubals." We were taking out normal uteruses as a way of sterilizing patients because in a Catholic hospital we weren't supposed to tie tubes. So a lot of hysterectomies were performed back then that were just tubals by another name. Then there were the times that the health of the patient demanded that we actually perform a tubal, and we had no other choice. That meant we had to do a song and dance for the bishop. In those cases we added a little paragraph in the operation notes that said, "After examining the patient and determining how attenuated the uterus had become from prior pregnancies we did not feel that it would support another pregnancy. In consequence, we isolated the uterus from the ovaries." What that meant was that we had tied the tubes. So we never did any tubals even when we did tubals; they were "uterine isolations." The bishop might have known what was going on. I wouldn't have been surprised. If he did, he kept it under his mitre.

My first major surgical case that second year was a patient we called Petite Patterson. The Petite Patterson case taught me as much as any other single case I ever had. Petite's real name was Michelle, but she got the nickname because she was a small woman who gained almost a hundred pounds in one year. She had been having really terrible periods and just couldn't stop putting on weight. Her abdomen was excessively protuberant and when I examined her I found a basketball-sized tumor in her pelvis. It felt like it might weigh a hundred pounds itself, and I was sure that it was cancer — she had all that pain and the huge mass looked semi-solid.

So we called up the oncologist. Second-years don't get cancer cases, but I got to stay on this one simply because it had come through the benign clinic and, until we were able to go in, Petite Patterson was considered only a possible cancer patient. I got to scrub with a chief (Val) and the oncologist. This particular oncologist shared my initials KK and was an outstanding operator. That was in part because he was obsessive-compulsive. I don't mean he acted as if he had obsessive-compulsive disorder; I mean he most definitely had it. KK made Ron Fishman look careless. Some of us had been to his house and upon discovering that he had alphabetized all the canned goods in his kitchen, we clearly had no choice but to remove the labels from all the cans. KK didn't find that nearly as amusing as we did.

We took Petite Patterson to the OR, and it took us thirteen hours to do the hysterectomy. When we went in, all the anatomy was brown because it had been dyed by bleeding from her endometriosis. She had a 35,000-cc tumor — benign endometrioma — and her entire abdomen was covered inside with smaller, chocolate-brown cysts. It was the worst case of endometriosis I have ever seen. Petite Patterson lost eighty-five pounds that day. Her weight gain had been all tumor. The disease had, as it often does, distorted many of the organs, structures, and tissues of the abdomen nearly beyond recognition. Disease distorts anatomy. That truth took me back to my med school anatomy class and Jan Negulesco. With enough of this sort of experience I could imagine myself in some distant day knowing human anatomy in the thorough and detailed way he did. I wasn't close to that day yet.

"Oh, what's this tubular structure here?"

"That's the urethra."

Removing what needs to come out in those circumstances is some of the most challenging surgical work that can be done. I did what I could at first, then KK took over in his slow, obsessively methodical way. Val spelled him sometimes, and sometimes he had something for me to do. We broke for lunch, worked, broke for dinner, and worked into the evening. I thanked Val and KK for letting me do as much as they did, and my thanks were heartfelt. Petite Patterson's case was a short, intense, and extremely valuable seminar in anatomy. I was limp with exhaustion when we were done, but I had learned more than a year's worth of normal hysterectomies would have taught me. The best part of it was that Petite Patterson recovered completely. A few days after the procedure she went home.

Since I'm discussing major gynecological procedures, it's worth talking about surgical technique and style here. When you're taking out an organ, you first need to identify the blood supply, then you must close each blood feeder separately and work your way around the organ until it's completely disconnected. At that point you can take it out. But do you take it out in one piece or do you dissect it? There's kind of a matter of pride involved with that question. Too many doctors, especially younger ones, want to take everything out in one piece. Sometimes that's impossible because the organ's taking up all the space around it. If you're prudent and experienced, you take part of it out, then some more, then some more. Work as you go. Some operators don't consider that elegant enough, however, and they'll try to take out everything in one piece. The pathologists certainly like that. They're not crazy about getting a uterus in four or five pieces because reassembling an organ for pathological inspection makes their job a little bit harder. Sometimes, though, that's just what you have to do. When I teach now, I often struggle with residents who try to take a uterus out in one piece for style points and spend an extra hour trying to do it. Every minute the patient is open is an opportunity for problems to start, whether from the procedure itself or from contamination. Get in, do a slick job, and get out. Don't worry about elegance. KK was one of the best operators I've ever seen and sometimes what he removed looked like a jigsaw puzzle.

Another of those second-year cases that taught me so much was a patient named Tammy Boyle. Tammy had a car accident at about twenty-two to twenty-four weeks and came in with a lot of abdominal pain right in front. We scanned her and decided that she had an anterior fibroid. We thought maybe she was cutting off the blood supply to the fibroid as her uterus grew and that was causing the pain. Over the course of our examination, she got scanned many, many times and we noticed that her baby didn't have much fluid around it and the fibroid never changed its appearance. As the pregnancy grew we became more concerned about the baby because of the small amount of fluid around it. We finally decided that we couldn't wait any longer and needed to induce the baby when she was about thirty-four weeks. We decided to do an amniocentesis to find out if the baby's lungs were mature, so we drew off some fluid and it came back immature. We waited a week and then induced labor.

During the labor the intern said, "Man, she's a tough cervical exam. I can barely get to the cervix. It's way up behind the pubic bone and it's not dilated at all. We've been giving her Pitocin all day long, and she's just not dilating."

That was the first time I had ever heard that description, but, like the story of the prolapsing fibroid, it has become one of those triggers that sets off alarm bells in my head. When you can't get the cervix to dilate you'd better start considering the possibility that the baby is not in the uterus.

Tammy never dilated so we decided to do a C-section. We took her back, opened her up, and there was a big, blue mass in her pelvis with a little tiny uterus sitting on top of it. The uterus was the thing we had been calling a fibroid, and the baby was behind the uterus in the broad ligament — that big, blue mass. We were stumped, but we knew who wouldn't be, so we called in Vic Fortin.

Vic took a look, pushed his glasses back on his head, and said, "I've seen three of these. An abdominal pregnancy. They're about one in twenty thousand births. Now, whatever you do, don't touch that placenta."

The placenta was embedded on the abdomen. It's not in the uterus, so if you remove the placenta there's nothing to clamp down on the huge blood supply meant for the baby. The patient will bleed to death and it won't take very long.

Now we knew that Vic had dealt with these before, but he wasn't scrubbed. The main doc who was scrubbed was a young attending — one of the hotshots. Vic left, and this guy started mucking around in there in a nerve-wracking way. He touched the placenta, just a little bit, and the patient started bleeding, a lot. He backed away, realized that he'd better follow Vic's advice, and managed to get the bleeding stopped. We tied off the placenta and left it in.

The baby had never been in the uterus so when we had done the amniocentesis we had just been sampling a little escaped fluid that happened to be around the baby. There was no amniotic sac. The baby had been constricted in an abnormal space so it had some problems with movement, but those cleared up and the baby girl ended up just fine. Although it was a rare and dangerous condition, the birth was relatively simple. The baby was right there when we opened up, and we never had to go into the uterus. We just left the placenta alone and hoped it would disintegrate. Over time it did to some degree, but eight months later we went in and took the remains out. That was a case for KK and his obsessive virtuosity, because that big, necrotic mass had made Tammy's anatomy hard to recognize.

It may seem surprising that even experienced doctors have problems identifying certain conditions. It's really not though. There's Vic Fortin-type experience in which you, literally, have seen everything and there's the more common amount of medical experience, and those doctors can get stumped. Because of the volume of work we second-years had, that period was one in which I saw a lot of the difficult cases that taught me a lot.

There was a University of Connecticut patient, Rose Dinovo, who came from a very small town and whose ob-gyn was following her for a cervical pregnancy. That's a type of ectopic pregnancy where the placenta implants on the cervix instead of in the uterus. The cervix is part of the uterus, but it's definitely not where the placenta should implant. Her doc had done an ultrasound at six or seven weeks and stuck on a note that said, "Low-lying placenta. Consider possibility of cervical pregnancy."

A cervical pregnancy is a kind of medical emergency because they usually only get to about seven or eight weeks before the patient either gets septic or begins to hemorrhage. So we were surprised to see another ultrasound record done at twelve weeks and that ultrasound had a note that said, "Cervical pregnancy confirmed. Consider clinical correlation." "Consider clinical correlation" is a radiology phrase that means, basically, "Do something!"

Rose's doctor was trying to get her pregnancy to viability which is about twenty-four to twenty-six weeks. That's simply impossible with a cervical pregnancy. None of us had heard of a cervical pregnancy getting beyond twelve weeks. So Rose's doctor called up U Conn when she was about eighteen weeks and was bleeding and told them,

"I have a patient here who's eighteen weeks and three days and she's having some bleeding with a cervical pregnancy."

The high-risk OB at U Conn said, "Well, she can't have a cervical pregnancy if she's eighteen weeks."

"Oh, no. I think she does," her doc said. "I was trying to get her about six more weeks, but it doesn't look like she's going to make it, so I need to transfer her to your hospital."

The U Conn guy, sensing an oncoming train wreck, didn't argue and just said, "Okay. Great. Send her to St. Francis. We'll take care of her there."

They sent her up by ambulance and she came into the ER where it's the second-year's job to evaluate patients. Small (Craig) was on duty, got the ultrasounds, read them, and thought that it certainly didn't look good, so he put a speculum in, looked, and the cervix was huge with an ominous mass behind it and a good amount of bleeding. Small called Val and the attending who happened to be the oncologist at U Conn — a hotshot, expert young surgeon, who was good, but who hadn't done OB for many years. He looked at the cervix and said, "There's no way that's a cervical pregnancy. You can't get to eighteen weeks with a cervical pregnancy. She's just having a miscarriage."

He took a ring forceps and pulled the mass out and Craig told me that it sounded like someone had turned on a bathtub faucet. Massive hemorrhaging. Luckily, they had a gynecological oncologist there on the team, so they were able to do a very quick emergency hysterectomy. She ended up getting fifty-six units of blood. You only have six units in your entire body. Mothers a little more. She bled out nine times her blood volume.

It had indeed been a cervical pregnancy and the surgeon had pulled out the placenta. Rose's physician had the correct diagnosis but was out to lunch on his treatment. The hotshot knew that the pregnancy wasn't viable but had no clue what it was or how to terminate it safely. The whole episode was another example of the uncomfortable paradox that often the most learning happens during the biggest screw-ups. Thank God Rose recovered.

That second year taught me more than just anatomy and operating skills. While dealing with more cases and more doctors than ever before, I also learned an uncomfortable truth about the politics of medicine, and Rose Dinovo's case touched on that. Doctors are not all on the same team. In a perfect world, certainly, they're all working for the good of the patient. Sometimes, though, other agendas get in the way and good physicians end up working at cross-purposes. The purest example of that is when doctors try to keep patients off their service and on someone else's.

Say a patient comes into the ER complaining of abdominal pain. She gets examined by the ER doc who suspects appendicitis and calls in a surgeon. The surgeon isn't sold on the diagnosis, though, and his floor is bursting with patients. He thinks it's more likely to be pelvic inflammatory disease (PID) so he calls in a gynecologist. When the gynecologist is done with her examination, she thinks that the ER doc is right and it's probably appendicitis. Her case load isn't any smaller than the surgeon's and that reality has the same influence on her that it had on him. The ER doc, for her part, wants the patient out of her ER, and rightly so. The other two have got to figure out what's wrong and do something about it. Consider clinical correlation!

Someone ends up taking the patient, of course, and most of the time the poor soul ends up on the appropriate service. I must confess, though, that there are few greater pleasures in medicine than finding out that your diagnosis was right and being able to rub it in with another physician. Imagine that after the kind of tug-of-war I've described you've had a patient kicked over to your service for PID and while you're doing a laparoscopy you find a sick appendix. You take a picture of it, lay it casually on a conference room table and then call the surgeon and ask him to stop around for a just a minute. Absolute joy. Of course, it happens the other way around, too, but let's not dwell on that.

Such are the dark truths of medicine. There are others and I'll get to them later. Learning these truths and learning the skills I needed to be the kind of doctor I wanted to be. That all started happening that second year. I was beginning to grow up as a physician, and I still had half of my residency to go.

Chapter 8

Growing Up

In Which Interns Learn to Rely on Me

The third year of the residency was when I began to feel like a real doctor. I was over the hump — senior to half the residents and supervisor of the new crop of interns. Now I was the lifeguard that Val had been to me in my internship and was finally feeling like I could run the show if I had to. I had, after all, been running the show at night throughout the second year. In addition to all those good things, I got four months to take elective courses in ob-gyn subspecialties. After an intern year filled with terror and a second year filled with work this year looked like fun.

It proved to be challenging fun. The electives were thirty-day crash courses on subspecialties in which I had little experience, such as newborn intensive care, maternal fetal medicine, oncology, and endocrine infertility. In the second year we did just general ob-gyn — six months of obstetrics and six months of gynecology — so these third-year electives were meant to get us up to speed in more complex and demanding areas of our field.

The surgery became more complex as well. Third-years did high-risk obstetrics such as pregnancies complicated by diabetes, hypertension, or birth defects. All the tough cases that came through the intern's clinic got bumped up to us. This was the year that I began doing vaginal hysterectomies; the "vag hyst" is the pinnacle of difficulty in gynecological surgery. All the hysterectomies I did up to this point were abdominal. We opened the abdomen and went in. In the vag hyst, we worked in the confines of the vagina and avoided the trauma of an incision. The anatomy that was literally open to us before was now accessible just through the narrow channel of the vagina. The procedure is far easier on the patient but far harder for her doctor.

I won't forget my first one. It was in the first few weeks of the year. We had just gotten a new attending, and I was scheduled to assist him. When we got to the scrub room he said, "Dr. Kington, how many vaginal hysterectomies have you performed?"

"Well, actually, none."

"How many have you assisted on?"

That was a little more comfortable. "Probably thirty, thirty-five."

"Then you'll do well handling this one by yourself. If you need my assistance, I'll be in the lounge."

Then he went out to the OR lounge, sat down, and read a newspaper.

I did do well, but that sort of sink-or-swim approach is not one that I admire. The attending's intentions were good, and his method wasn't unusual. Getting thrown in the deep end was fairly common in those days before litigation became an everyday presence. Today, an attending sitting in the lounge during a procedure is considered grounds for dismissal.

That's an interesting discussion, though. Sink-or-swim shortens the learning curve, no doubt about it — and a confident, experienced doctor is what a medical education is supposed to produce. "See one; do one; teach one" is a cliché with a long history in medicine (even though it grossly simplifies the reality). I don't see a need for an either/or approach. I give my residents a lot of independence, and I know it's good for them and the patients. Even so, I'm still glad that the days of storing your attending down the hall are over. The dangerous weak link in sink-or-swim is that sometimes the resident doesn't *know* when things are going wrong. The young doctor might be confident and competent, but things can go south in a hurry and sometimes that's not immediately apparent.

In a vaginal hysterectomy, for instance, you have to find a layer that's very thin between the bladder and the uterus. If you go too low, you start cutting into the uterus and if you go too high, you start cutting into the bladder. You don't know you're too high until you see urine spilling. You don't know you're too low until you find yourself trying to figure out where you are in the abdomen when you're not in the abdomen at all.

You're also flying blind when you're going up the side of the uterus and clamping vessels. You're trying to get to the point where the ovaries are attached to the uterus because you're going to cut and clamp those vessels. You have to get around to the top of the uterus and you can't see a thing, so it's completely a matter of feel. It's a tricky situation. Once when I was a second assistant on a vaginal hysterectomy, the med student was holding a bunch of instruments attached to the end of the uterus. It was almost out. We only had one more pedicle (artery and vessel) to go — up there on the top. Then, without tugging very hard at all, the med student delivered the uterus. We never got a clamp on that last vessel so there was a flood of bleeding and the vessel snapped back into the abdomen like a rubber band and was gone. We had to do a laparotomy to tie it off. Those are deep waters to be sinking or swimming in, and I'm glad that the way my first vag hyst experience occurred could no longer happen.

I did swim, though, and once I learned the procedure I started culling the chief's clinic for all the vaginal hysterectomies I could find — so I got good at them in a hurry. One of my greatest surgical coups that year was finding six Spanish-speaking vag-hyst patients. That meant that I was able to do all their surgery and because I didn't speak Spanish one of my unfortunate second-years, who did, had to do all the rounds on them. Perfect.

Third year was memorable as well because of all that new technology that was coming along. St. Francis got a new ultrasound machine that cost a quarter of a million dollars. Thirty years ago I would have used an exclamation point after that price. Not anymore. It was an impressive machine. We had never seen images that clear and useful. One of my duties that year was to follow our ultrasonographers which I found highly valuable. I learned a lot about the visual aspects of diagnosis, and though I wasn't close to the diagnostic instincts of Vic Fortin, I was getting better case by case. Today we have 3D machines that provide far better images, but that new ultrasound machine at St Francis was a huge help in diagnosing all sorts of problems. Imagine trying to learn from a book illustrated with blurry, primitive woodcuts, then suddenly being able to use one with photographs. I was lucky to have that wonderful machine to learn on. Sometimes getting a late career start works in your favor.

Those electives were probably the best aspect of that whole year. I got to work with subspecialists who were experts in their fields. A residency, of course, is simply a continuation of the doctor's education that begins in medical school, and there were times in that third year when I was learning things at a rate that reminded me of med school. Each elective was for thirty days and the resident was assigned to the subspecialty during the day.

The setup was that there was an attending, who was the subspecialist, and a fellow, who was a recent graduate of the residency program and was going through a fellowship in that subspecialty. Then there was me, the outsider resident, and even though I was third in importance there was a lot to learn just by watching and listening. Nights remained the same. Third-years still took call in their department to back up the interns.

Endocrine Infertility was my first elective. Just as with ultrasonography, the field was being transformed by technology. A whole range of possibilities for infertile patients was now possible, including in-vitro fertilizations. We helped a lot of couples conceive who could never have done so a few years earlier and that was very satisfying. Being around the joy of birth was one of the reasons I chose ob-gyn in the first place, and now I was able to be one of the docs who could make it happen for people who had no hope before. Wonderful.

In the very early days of in-vitro, however, it wasn't covered by insurance companies. So we dealt with patients who were wealthy enough to pay for the procedure themselves. That introduced us to what we called "the Greenwich set," and they were a whole different type of patient.

One case from the Greenwich set involved a very rich couple who had been going through a long and expensive process to have a baby. I came in on the tail end of a months-long process. He'd had a semen analysis and she'd had a uterine analysis and everything looked normal, but nothing was working. My infertility attending sat them down and told them, "I know you've done all those tests, but we can't find a reason for your infertility, so we need to run a post-coital test. You'll have sex, then come in for testing two to eight hours later, and we'll examine the semen and the cervical mucus. That might be able to tell us something that we're not catching with the other tests, because 40 percent of the time the man is the cause and 40 percent of the time the woman is. The other 20 percent of the time it's the combination of the two and that's what we can find out with post-coital testing."

The wife was very willing and the husband far less so, but she prevailed and they came in for their test. The results were interesting to say the least. There was no sperm in the cervical mucus.

The attending had the husband in for a conference and showed him the results of the previous tests. They said normal sperm count and normal motility. Then he showed him the coital test results that said no sperm present. Then he just sat there. Finally, the husband admitted to us that, despite probably fifty thousand dollars spent in the workup for infertility, he'd had a vasectomy before their marriage and didn't want his wife to know. She had wanted kids and he pretended that he did. The whole charade had been, apparently, in hopes that she would become discouraged and give up trying. The million-dollar question, of course, was where the husband got the semen for the all the fertility tests. It turned out to be from a friend. Now, *that's* a friend.

The husband was stuck, but we were, too, in a way. Because of patient confidentiality rules, we couldn't tell the wife the truth. All we could do was tell her the test results and hope that she put two and two together. What a betrayal of trust and love. I've always wondered how that story ended.

I wish I could say that that sort of betrayal was unique in my experience, but actually I had seen something just as bad way back in med school. One of the attendings had been treating a young woman who had had a sex change operation and refused to tell her fiancé. The sex reassignment surgery had been a great success. She was a very beautiful young woman and was outwardly indistinguishable from any woman to the doctors who examined her. She refused to tell her partner, though. What a potentially destructive decision that was. The things we do for love.

Another odd case during the Endocrine Fertility elective happened at the opposite end of the income range from the Greenwich couple. We had a young woman who was pregnant — infertility wasn't the problem — but who had no idea who the father was. She lived in a commune and had had sex with thirty different men in close proximity to when she conceived. She wanted us to do some genetic testing so that she could figure out who the father was before the pregnancy got too far along. My elective month was over before I found out what happened to her. I wonder if she told the father and if she had the baby.

After the month in one elective I cycled back into the regular routine for another two months or so then on to another elective. I got to go back to the Midwest for the Maternal Fetal Medicine elective. I was excited about working at Ohio State under their new chair Steve Peters, a doctor who was at the top of his field. Peters was a big deal. He was published all over the place, was a rising star in Maternal Fetal Medicine, and I was thinking about next year, my chief's year, when I would be applying for jobs — probably including Ohio State. So, flying out to Columbus, I read all of Peters's articles. I wanted to be able to impress him if the opportunity came up by quoting from something he wrote. The opportunity, of course, never even remotely presented itself. He never mentioned one of the articles in the month that I was there. It was worth reading the papers from an educational standpoint and that was one of my favorite and most useful electives. From an impress-the-boss standpoint, though, I might as well have memorized his license plate number.

One of the things I remember most strongly about that month in Columbus was moving in with my parents. At age thirty-six I can tell you that was a very strange experience. Don't get me wrong. My parents were terrific people. It just was not what I expected. When I was growing up, they had been live wires, and with six siblings the house was always loud and full of life. My dad was from Oklahoma, was a star athlete in high school, and went directly from his graduation into the Marines. It was right after Pearl Harbor and when he finished boot camp they made him a drill instructor himself — two weeks after he joined. I'm sure that all our military training courses were accelerated then, but that's still a good indication of the kind of guy he was. He fought in the Pacific and was wounded in the Marshall Islands. It was a friendly fire incident; an American soldier shot him from behind. He always said with traditional Marine disdain that he had been "shot in the ass by the U.S. Army." It saved his life. While he was in the hospital his unit was sent on to Okinawa where it suffered 150% casualties. Even the reinforcements were killed. The only two survivors from his unit were Dad and a double amputee.

When he got out of the service he started working for a loan company, Dial Finance, and worked his way up through the company. We lived all over the country as he went from office to office and he ended up on Dial's board — the only one who wasn't a member of the founder's family.

Mom was just as vital a person. She was interested in everything, was a great conversationalist, read like crazy, raised all those kids, and was still downhill skiing in her eighties.

Those were the parents I knew, so it was very odd that things around their house were deadly dull. I don't know what I had expected from them in their mid-seventies but having grown up with the noise and craziness of six siblings, it was striking to see how quiet and regular their lives had become. They had their drink before dinner, ate, then sat around and read or talked. No TV. No noise. In a way it was relaxing after a day at the hospital, but it got old very quickly and it really brought home to me how much pressure and challenge had become my norm. I loved spending that month with my parents, but on the return flight to Hartford I was really looking forward to getting back to Nancy, our lively house full of kids, and the fray of St. Francis.

The next elective came along a couple of months later — oncology. It was my least favorite of all the subspecialties I studied because, first of all, it was oncology, and also because of the odd professional politics that got in the way. Oncology has always dogged me in my career. I have always found cancer medicine depressing, have always tried to minimize my time doing it, and have never been able to avoid it. At St. Francis we didn't have any officially required electives, but everyone took oncology so I was stuck. The rotation was done at the University of Connecticut hospital because they had a lot more oncology cases out there.

The problem was that there's a residency program at UConn, so I was inserted as an outsider into their Oncology service. I showed up the first day for rounds and the chief resident asked me who I was.

"I'm Kevin Kington from St. Francis. I'm starting my oncology elective today."

"Oh. Oh, yeah. Well, we've got twelve patients on our Gyn Oncology service in these twelve rooms, so we'd like you to round on all of them every morning."

It was a pretty heavy workload, and I thought that I should get there early each morning. So I started my rounds about 5:30. I looked at every patient — and these were sick patients — and I took vitals, asked questions, and wrote it down, and by 7:30 I was ready for morning report. But I noticed that every time that I had left a room there had been a UConn third-year going in after me. I got to morning report and the chief asked who was going to report on the patient in room 211. I said, "Well, I can."

She said, "No, I think our third-year is going to present her." So their third-year, the one trailing me on my rounds, presented the patient, talked about all the information that I had collected, and described what was going to be done in the treatment. Next patient; same thing. We went through the entire morning report, and I didn't say a word. Everything I had done was duplicated by their resident and she got the floor. I was, basically, being treated like a medical student.

The service had two fellows, a chief resident, a third-year, and then me and the pecking order was becoming clearer and clearer. So I went to the chief and said, "I really want to feel a part of this team, so if I'm going to round on patients I don't see why another third-year should duplicate everything I'm doing."

"No. No. We have to do that," she said. "The oncologists want our third-year to round on all the patients."

"Well, do I have to round on them, then, if it's just going to be done by someone else? Can't I just go with your person and watch her round and I'll learn just as much?"

"Hmm. Okay."

About the third day of the rotation one of the oncologists called me into his office and said, "Kevin, you know you've got two fellows in front of you; you've got a chief in front of you and a UConn third-year in front of you. So I don't think you're going to get too much surgery on weekdays. I was wondering if you wanted to scrub for our cases on Thanksgiving and the next day." That meant the emergency cases because that's all that was scheduled for those off-days.

"So," I said, "I'm going to be here for thirty days but the only days I'm actually going to be able to work are Thanksgiving and Thanksgiving Friday."

"Yeah," he said. "I guess that's about it."

I wouldn't get to do rounds. I wouldn't get to do surgery. So I started showing up about 10:30 and going home about 3:00. That was a wasted month. Thank God it was oncology.

I did learn a valuable fashion tip that month, though. One of the oncologists was a meticulous dresser and made a comment to the chief one day about a patient's visitor.

"Look at that buffoon. His shoes don't even match his belt!"

Looking down at my black belt and brown shoes I suppose I should have felt sheepish, but I didn't. I just chalked it up to working with Easterners.

A dud elective like the UConn oncology rotation could happen, but generally the courses were terrifically useful, and in one case that I know of, life changing. And I was there to see that happen in my second Maternal Fetal Medicine rotation. The program's fellow was a very smart young doctor, John DeArmond, and one day we were sitting in the office with the attending, Tony Vintzileos, when the phone rang. John answered, and it was a reporter from the *Hartford Courant.*

"There's been an outbreak of Fifth Disease in the Torrington school system," she said. "Do you know what Fifth Disease is?"

John was mildly annoyed. "Yeah, I know what Fifth Disease is."

That's a rash-causing parvovirus that's fairly common among schoolchildren, but historically not as common as four of the other rash-causers: measles, rubella, scarlet fever, and Dukes' disease. Thus the name.

The reporter continued, "They have eight pregnant teachers in the schools there who think they've been exposed to Fifth Disease. Is that a problem?"

John covered the mouthpiece and leaned toward Tony.

"Some reporter's calling about Fifth Disease. Sounds all worried that some pregnant teachers were exposed to it. There's no problem with that and pregnancy is there? Maybe I'll just tell her not to worry about it."

Tony Vintzileos looked at him and said, "Do you really think you should risk your entire career by giving a flippant answer to a newspaper about Fifth Disease and its relationship to pregnancy when we don't know anything about it?"

John reddened a bit. "No, I probably shouldn't."

"Why don't you put off the reporter for a little while," Tony said. "Maybe we've found the subject of your fellowship thesis."

So John told the reporter that there wasn't much information on the subject but that he'd look into it and get back to her. The next day John went up to Torrington, which is just over Avon Mountain from Hartford, and interviewed all those teachers. Then he brought them in to the hospital for ultrasounds. The more he worked, the more he found, and he became the discoverer of the relationship between parvovirus B19 and pregnancy. It turned out that it is, indeed, a big problem. The teachers who were in their first trimester had a bad prognosis for their pregnancies; the lucky ones in their third trimester were better off. John found that Fifth Disease in a pregnant woman who hasn't had it before crosses the placenta and causes aplastic anemia in the fetus and increases the risk of heart failure for the fetus.

John saved the third trimester babies with transfusions, and that discovery and therapy became his career. When John finished his fellowship, he began to speak around the world about the dangerous relationship between Fifth Disease and pregnancy. His work has saved countless babies; he's become the guru of parvovirus B19; and I was there listening in when fate made its telephone call.

Third year was not just electives. The routine went on — lots of deliveries, C-sections, hysterectomies, and various surgeries. The hardest part about being a third-year was riding herd on the interns. They don't know what they're doing at first and so the third-years are basically covering the whole house by themselves (and sometimes, as in Val's case, getting called in the middle of the night about giving a patient Tylenol). The first six months are pretty brutal, but then the interns start to get their sea legs and things calm down.

I lucked out with my interns. They were a good batch, and one — Mark Kent — was outstanding. Mark had an unusual background. He grew up on Guam and was schooled at the University of Hawaii. Most of the residents at St. Francis came from the Eastern Corridor. I was considered an exotic specimen for having come from the Midwest (faraway land of black belts and brown shoes). So Mark was unique. He was naturally curious, a quick learner, and ended up being very good at a lot of things, including auto mechanics and sailing. When he was fourteen years old, he sailed his fourteen-foot boat from Guam to Japan. His mother might have objected, but she didn't find out until he got there.

Mark was unusually accomplished, but he was still an intern with the intern's combination of book smarts, practical ignorance, and abject terror. Early that year he called me at home and told me that he thought he had a clinic patient with a ruptured ectopic pregnancy. I was suddenly looking into a mirror. All the memories from my first year came back of trying to roust J.B. out of his house for a ruptured ectopic and of his ill-fated culdocentesis.

"What are the symptoms, Mark?"

He ran through some scary stuff, then said, "She's lost so much blood that her eyelids are white."

That seemed like an odd yet insightful observation, and I told him I would be right in. When I got there the patient was in bad shape. I thought she was Caucasian when she rolled by, then realized with a shock that she was a black woman and had lost so much blood that her skin had no color. We got her into the ER, got the bleeding stopped, and transfused her. It was a close call, but she made it. Watching Mark that night was a small rite of passage for me. Having faced the same situation as an intern two years before, I could recognize his fear, and I could sense his relief at having me there. It was a nice feeling to be on the other side of the anxiety. The aura of competence is a valuable tool for a doctor. Mark picked it up that night and it gave him confidence. At times throughout my career I've had residents tell me that they breathed a sigh of relief when they had an emergency and I walked through the door. They always said that I seemed so calm.

I would never tell them that there were plenty of times I was racing through possibilities in my head and thinking, "What the hell do I do about *this*?" If methodical comes off as unflappable that's okay with me. So working with Mark that night was really satisfying. It was good, too, to work with an intern who I could tell was absorbing everything that was happening.

A few weeks later we worked another case together, and Mark got some experience with some of the more unusual surgery that an ob-gyn does. He also got some experience with the competition that can flare up between doctors in different fields. Mark and I were on one night; he was covering labor and delivery and I got called in to do a C-section for a clinic patient. We were getting ready to start, but, as usual, the anesthesia was delayed. We always had problems with the anesthesia at St. Francis and that was not unusual back then. Now things are very different, as I'm sure they are there, too. But in those days the anesthesiologists worked in the OR with the surgeons and they kind of saw epidurals and C-sections as a distraction that they didn't want to deal with. Especially epidurals. They'd have to leave the surgery floor, come up to give the epidural, and then stay with the patient to monitor her progress. It turned into an antagonistic relationship because we were always trying to get the epidurals for our patients and they were always dragging their feet. That night the anesthesiologist finally got there, and he was making his excuses.

"We had a hot appendix downstairs. Well, we thought it was an appendix and then it turned out not to be."

Curious, I asked him "Then what was it?"

"It was an ovarian mass in a twelve-year-old girl."

"An ovarian mass?" I said. "Didn't the surgeons want to talk to us about that?"

"Oh, you know surgeons," he said. "They know how to take out an ovary and they're not going to call you about that."

So Mark and I did the C-section and the next morning we were at breakfast. (In those days you didn't get any rest time after you were on call all night.) The surgeons were at the next table and I could hear the chief resident talking about the procedure from the night before.

I turned around and I said, "You guys taking out ovaries now, are you?"

With the typical surgeon's machismo he said, "What? You think we don't know how to take out an ovary? We can do hysterectomies, too." His people all laughed.

"I'm sure you can," I said, "But weren't you a little reluctant to take an ovary out of a twelve-year-old girl?"

He got kind of quiet and said, "Why? Is that a problem?"

"Well, yeah, it is. Twelve-year-old girls usually don't have ovarian cysts unless it's cancer."

He went silent.

"You'd better talk to the gyn oncologist about that case," I said, and Mark and I got up and left for the OR.

We had to get upstairs to a case of a thirty-three-year-old woman with a dermoid — a benign cyst of the ovary. As we went up the elevator I went into my teaching mode with Mark telling him about the peculiarities of dermoids. The tumor can generate all sorts of unusual things inside it — teeth, hair, different kinds of tissue. They can be malignant as well, in which case they often have brain tissue. I told him that once we got this one out we ought to go to the pathology lab and take a look at it. He'd learn a lot about their composition.

So after we finished we found the pathologist and I said, "We came in to look at that dermoid."

He interrupted with, "Yeah! That's a really interesting case! It's got brain tissue in it and hair and ..."

Now I interrupted him. "Wait a minute. You said it has brain tissue?"

"Oh, yeah."

"So it was malignant?!"

"Oh, sure. It's malignant."

I couldn't believe it, and it turned out that he wasn't talking about our dermoid. He was talking about that young girl's ovarian cyst. That's how we found out that it was malignant — later than we would have if the surgeon hadn't decided that he was a gyn oncologist.

That patient was in big trouble; she was dead in a year. Finding out twelve hours later didn't make any difference in her survival. The malignancy would have been found out eventually through procedural channels, but that's not the point. The point was that it was sloppy work on a life-or-death case caused by professional hubris. Mark had never seen that kind of turf battle. An intern learns all sorts of things, though, and I tried to communicate to him the importance of training yourself not to go beyond your expertise and abilities. That can be very hard to do. General ob-gyns train with gyn oncologists and participate in all sorts of procedures. They still need to step back when they can and let the expert do it, even if they know they could do a good job themselves. Because, again, it's those situations where you don't even know that things are going wrong that are the killers. Just call for help. It's better for the patient and it's one of the most important things you learn in a residency.

The other side of that coin is that sometimes you don't have time to call for help and you have to keep your head and move forward. There was another of my interns that third year that I'll call Angela. She was serious about her work and she ended up being a good resident, but one case early that year really tested her. It was another ruptured ectopic pregnancy. (If you're starting to think that ruptured ectopics are dangerous icebergs in the seas of gynecology, you're right.) This one was a type of ectopic that I had never seen myself — a cornual pregnancy. The pregnancy was in the muscular part of the uterus, called the cornu, or horn. It's especially dangerous because that's the thinnest part of the uterus and the pregnancy can cause the entire uterus to split open. When we opened the patient it looked like her blood was coming through a hose. Angela froze. She didn't speak, and she couldn't move for what seemed to me like an hour — though certainly it was just a minute. I took a clamp and clamped the uterus.

"Angela, we're going to have to take this uterus out. You're going to have to help me here."

Finally, she twitched. "But we can't! We didn't tell her we were going to do that."

"I know," I said, "But we've got no choice. She's going to lose her uterus. That's on the consent form. We need to move. Let's get going."

That being my first cornual ectopic, I wasn't the calmest person around either. But I was functioning. That's the difference a couple of years makes. Once I talked her off the ledge, Angela did a good job. But that's one of the other crucial things young doctors need to learn: how they'll react when the bottom falls out. There are times when you realize very simply that you're it. It's only you. You're the single thing between a patient and death. Get going.

Crisis management — specialized study — getting comfortable with major responsibility. The third year is a full one.

One of its primary jobs, of course, is getting the doctor ready to run things as a chief. I felt that I was ready for the fourth year and ready to take my place at that big table in the morning near John Gibbons and Vic Fortin. The idea seemed both very much earned and unbelievable at the same time. That double view was true of how my time as a resident felt, too — endless while I was doing it and dizzyingly fast in retrospect.

"My time" in the residency program, of course, wasn't just mine. It was shared by, and fueled by, Nancy and the kids. I haven't mentioned the family much so far in these chapters, but they are there on every page for me and in every moment of the quest to become a doctor. As a very private person, Nancy hasn't felt comfortable about showing up here in black and white for all to see. Nancy graciously agreed to help me describe the last year in the program. It was the final hurdle before I began private practice, and it was Nancy who made it possible for me to get here and that's not an exaggeration, either. Nancy worked as hard as I did every step of the way, and for her the move to Connecticut was a far bigger deal than it was for me. I had moved twenty times before I went away to college as our family followed my father's job around the country. I was used to being a gypsy. (On the last of those moves, from Cleveland to Columbus, I started at my new high school and met Nancy.)

Nancy, on the other hand, had moved once when she was six months old from New Lexington, Ohio, to Columbus. That's where all her memories were. Except for her one sister near Hartford, that's where all her family was. She was a little uneasy about the move.

I had never needed neighbors before, though I've always loved having them. We enjoyed our neighbors, but I never had to rely on them. When we came to Hartford suddenly I did, and we became very close. The kids were two, four, six, eight, and ten. Ginny and Patrick were too young for school and so they spent the day at home with me. Then at a school get-together, I met a new neighbor who had just moved there and she had two daughters whose ages fit right in with Ginny and Katie. We just clicked. She was a teacher who needed somebody to do before-and-after-school care, so I started watching her girls. Then it snowballed. One of the other neighbor parents had a day care service so I learned all the licensing rules for Connecticut from her: how many children you could supervise, what their ages could be — all the legal requirements. I ended up starting a little day care business. I put a small ad in the neighborhood paper, and then the word got out at the hospital and there were a lot of doctors' wives who wanted a day or two of child care. It worked well, and it was an interesting experience for me to be a mom and a businesswoman at the same time. I could contribute financially, and it didn't take any of my time away from our kids.

Besides the neighbors, the other thing I loved about Hartford was the quality of the schools. When we were planning the move we talked about putting the kids in Catholic schools, but the public schools in West Hartford were just so good that we couldn't pass that up. The summer programs were outstanding. Tim took summer classes and Emily and Katie had parts in summer plays. It was wonderful.

Nancy is right about the neighbors. We did have great ones and I'm so glad because, especially during the intern year, I arrived home from work completely useless. About all I could do was sleep. Nancy could have been very isolated, but our neighbors made the difference. We were still very much outsiders. Foreigners. This was the East, after all. You're really not a Connecticut native if your family got there in the past century. Our neighbors were terrific people, and they helped make a tough time easier. Nancy shares that perspective.

Looking back, we were so young. Thirty-three. We have four kids older than that now. Kevin was gone a lot and, yes, when he was home he was often just worn out. But the most important thing that we decided when we started this whole journey was that no matter how tough things got we would never wish the time away. We would never try to ignore the present and wait for the future. We wanted to enjoy the journey. And we did. Even the hard parts. That was just life.

For Nancy, one of the hardest parts about leaving home besides leaving her family was leaving behind our pediatrician, Dr. Klamar. He was kind of a god, and it was useful for me to see what kind of impact a physician can have on a family's life. I was always amused (and maybe a little jealous) at the weight that his opinion carried with Nancy. When one of the kids was sick I gave my diagnosis and opinion, but still anxious, Nancy would call Dr. Klamar. Then he would tell her the same thing that I had said, and Nancy would put down the phone with complete relief and say, "I feel so much better!" So with no Dr. Klamar around, and often with no Dr. Kington around, Nancy did beautifully. I couldn't have succeeded otherwise.

Patrick, our two-year-old son, had some of the most significant anxiety about the move, but we didn't find that out for a year or so. When we first got to Hartford, the house next door was being rebuilt because it had exploded. A gas leak from the septic system met up with a spark from an appliance and the explosion leveled the house. No one was hurt, but Patrick nursed a quiet fear about gas explosions for a long time until one day he asked us, "You know when the house next door exploded? Which one of 'em had gas?"

If your biggest fears are that size, you're doing pretty well. We had come to Connecticut wary of the move, missing Ohio, and thinking that there was no question about going back to Columbus when the residency was over. By the beginning of my last year we had started to think about staying.

Chapter 9

Chief Resident? Me?

In Which Power Does Not Corrupt

June became July, my third year was over, and I (along with Craig and Tony) was a chief resident. Those green interns Small, Medium, and Large were now the guys running things on the floor, and a license and private practice were in sight. It would have been satisfying to walk into a big office, put my feet up on an impressive desk, and relish the accomplishment. As usual, though, there was no time. There was no big office, either — just the same conference and on-call rooms in which I had sweated, learned, argued, and tried to catch sleep since I got to St. Francis. Everything else, though, had changed. As a chief, I was now primarily a teacher and administrator. My OB workload wasn't close to what it was in the third year. Chiefs decided which residents got which procedures, but it was considered bad form to cherry pick things for yourself, so all the interesting stuff went to the third-years. I assisted the residents who needed guidance and was paired with the second-year in the usual year-skipping mentoring scheme. Now I took calls from home, though. I felt like a big deal, but I didn't really care for it because I wasn't working with patients enough. I also discovered that, despite my newfound authority, my ability to change the way we did things in the department was severely limited.

When Craig, Tony, and I were finishing up our third year and getting ready to be chiefs we had some grand ideas about ways to revamp the residency program. We thought of the difficulties and frustrations we had faced as younger residents and, like good doctors, tried to figure out remedies. The biggest problem, we felt, was communication within the chain of command. The way we communicated responsibilities and expectations to one another within the department had become inefficient and so the formalities of rounding on patients and teaching residents had become sloppy. In short, who was responsible for what at which time wasn't always clear. Our changes meant that some attendings would have had to work a little harder and document decisions a little more carefully than they had been.

So right at the top of the fourth year we asked for a meeting with the department poohbahs to discuss our ideas. That was an eye-opener. I had thought that John Gibbons and Vic Fortin ran the residency program and didn't realize the weight that some of the older attendings carried. I didn't even know that they were involved at all. Well, they were.

There were three attendings at the meeting in addition to Gibbons and Fortin. The most vocal was Ronny DeArmond.

Ronny was fond of a sweater with a huge eagle on the front. So to the residents Ronny became The Eagle, with more than a little symbolism going on there. Ronny was a strong personality. He sat in our meeting, listened to what we had to say, took our written suggestions, read them quietly, then folded them and slid them into his nice leather notebook.

"Okay, here's what we're going to do this year."

What followed sounded a lot like what we had done every year before and that was pretty much that for our changes.

It interested me to see John Gibbons, the master politician, during all this. He had read our position paper and seemed open to the suggestions but gave the floor to Ronny and watched him cut us down to size. That was vintage Gibbons. He wasn't a devious man, but he wanted to please the attendings while maintaining his role as the demanding but fair father figure. Using Ronny as a hatchet man maintained both the status quo that his attendings wanted and a good relationship with his new chiefs.

I was starting to learn about the power structure of hospitals and what got my attention was the hidden power of those attendings. There's the acknowledged chain of command in any hospital that you can see in the staff directory, and then there is the hidden power with its roots in personalities, in admiration and retribution, in friendships, loyalties, rivalries, debts, and fears. That's the way of the world in any organization. It's just useful to realize that the serious business, altruism, and noble intentions of medicine don't put its institutions above the fray.

My own power relationships as a newbie chief were giving me problems in those first months, and the best illustration of that was the helipad incident. St. Francis was growing, and the hospital decided to build a helipad to give Life Flights direct access. It was a great idea and people were cranked up about it, especially the trauma surgeons. There was a lot of education going on about how to use the helipad, like how to get to it from your unit; what to wear when you got there; what your job was in getting the patient out of the chopper. The problem was that the education was centered on the emergency and trauma staffs. Along with a lot of other departments, the OBs weren't included in the orientation.

So around early fall of that year while I was still learning the job, I decided to go to lunch with Nancy and the kids. It was a pretty Saturday afternoon and we went to a Pizza Hut across the Connecticut River from the hospital. I had just settled into the booth when my beeper went off. I got on the restaurant phone and found out that there was a patient coming in by Life Flight. The nurse gave me quick details. The woman had experienced a crushing headache, went blind, then fell down and had a seizure. She was also eight months pregnant. It was a private patient and her attending was thirty minutes away. On a dangerous and complicated case like that I had to be there.

So I rushed out of the Pizza Hut, pointed the car back toward the bridge and floored it. As I sped across the river I heard the loud beating of the chopper and saw it slant dramatically right above the bridge. It was a classic movie moment and my pulse quickened. I kept the pedal to the metal and it was a weekend, so traffic was light. I was going to make it.

The problems started when I got to the hospital and realized that I really didn't know how to get to the helipad. I knew roughly where it was, but I didn't know the best lot to park in or the best entrance and elevator to take. Those are all the things that you learn in training. So I winged it. I knew which building the pad was on and I had seen the chopper come in, so I knew which end of the roof I needed. I found the elevator to the helipad, but I also found that it took a special key which no one had talked to us about. I ran over to the ER, grabbed the first white coat I saw.

"Where's the trauma surgeon on call? I need to get to the helipad."

"Oh, you can't go up there! Only people with the key can go up there!"

"I know! I need the guy with the key!"

So I found a maintenance guy with the key. Cliff took his own sweet time moseying over to the elevator. We headed for the roof. We got out.

Cliff said, "You've got to put on ear protectors and overalls. They're locked in this closet over here. I suppose you don't have a key for that, either, huh?"

I told him I didn't, and Cliff wasn't very happy about unlocking the closet for someone who didn't have the key. I don't know what to call that sort of thing. The psychology of exclusivity?

Or was it just the classic case of the person with a little bit of power? I was one of the people that the elevator and gear were being reserved *for*, but here was this guy trying to protect it all from being used. I guess that if the keys started to get used too much then the role of key keeper wasn't as important.

My impatience was starting to turn to anger and I'm a big guy. He finally got the closet unlocked. We put on the protective gear and went up under the spinning rotor of the chopper. It was loud and confused and bordering on a fiasco up there. One look at the patient made it clear that she was in bad shape — unconscious and posturing like a stroke victim. We got her down to the ER, and I did an ultrasound on the baby while everyone else was working on the mother. It was basically a code blue because at that point she had stopped breathing. The baby's heartbeat was all over the place. Since it was eight months I knew it was a viable child, but it was in distress. We had to act quickly.

So we called a neurosurgeon in and when he got there he just leaned against the wall with his arms folded watching the rest of us. That fit, I'm sorry to say, with my stereotype of neurosurgeons as odd people. I went over and engaged the wall prop in conversation.

"What do you think? Are you going to operate on this lady?"

"I dunno."

"Her baby's not looking too good. It needs to be delivered."

"I can't help you," the wall prop said. "I won't know whether she needs surgery until the CAT scan team gets here, and they're on call from home. I don't know if it's a bleed or if it's a clot."

This was frustrating and I said, "Well, can you make a guess? Where are you going with this?"

"I won't be able to tell you anything for half an hour."

The chaotic room was filled with crisis-mode professionals performing CPR, racing to start IVs and antibiotics, trying to save two lives.

I told the unmoved neurosurgeon that I would meet him in CAT scan in thirty minutes.

I got the patient out of there, called up to Labor and Delivery and told them we were going to do a stat C-section so be ready to roll immediately. What happened next was a perfect illustration of how fast rumors travel in a hospital. I got on the elevator went up to the fourth floor, got off, went to my unit, and after that amount of time — maybe two minutes — the unit coordinator found me.

"I hear you had an argument with the neurosurgeon."

I said, "What are you talking about?"

"Yeah," she said, "I heard that you said you were going to sacrifice the mother and save that baby!"

"I didn't tell him any such thing. We did have a few words, but that was all. Now let's go get this baby."

I've mentioned the dancelike quality of a good surgery and that's what the next twenty minutes were like. Little talking; quick, effective movements; everyone doing a part they knew instinctively. Soon we had a little red bawling girl in our hands. We got that C-section done in record time and got the mother down to CAT scan inside that half-hour window. As we rolled in one door the scan team was coming in another. It was perfect timing.

The neurosurgeon stared at the patient and said, "Did you just operate on this woman?"

It's hard to act nonchalant when you're out of breath, but I think I managed. "Oh. Sure. You said we had thirty minutes."

He looked at me for a few seconds then just shook his head. The great thing was that I got to scrub for the brain surgery. The CAT scan had shown that she had an arterioveinous malformation on her brain — a congenital bundle of vessels that had bled. We had to go in and clip that off. I wouldn't have been able to do neurosurgery any other year but my fourth, so that was one time that being a chief got me some valuable hands-on work. Three months later, that patient walked out of the hospital with her baby.

That was the first time the hospital had ever used the helipad and the results were as good as they possibly could be for the patient, but it was clear that the training procedures had to be sharpened and expanded to all the surgical specialties, including OB. I made that part of my job during the fourth year. This incident also pointed up one of the crucial roles of the chief. Because of the way that the hospital departments were structured and because of the inconsistent ways of communicating that Tony, Craig, and I had tried to fix, chiefs were the only real liaison between the residents of different departments. Interns seldom talked to those in other departments and second and third years had to go through the chief. Consultations happened either chief-to-chief, attending-to-attending, or not at all.

Besides being a liaison, I wrote schedules, taught procedures, bailed out the overwhelmed, reassured the discouraged, and disciplined the slackers. The problem children were rare, but I had to crack the whip occasionally. There was one intern who would disappear while he was on call. He wouldn't answer his pages, and no one could find him in the call rooms. He had probably found the perfect place to sleep. We never discovered it, so it must have been a lulu. It was my job to make it clear to him that his work ethic needed to be at the same level as his ingenuity. He shaped up, but he never really lived down his reputation and got ragged for it from then on. After a couple of years in private practice, I came back for the chief's dinner they threw for this guy and there were some oversized, hilariously brutal pictures of him holed up in obscure parts of the hospital wearing the red and white "Where's Waldo" hat. His parents were dinner guests and it was uncomfortable. But medical people have long memories and tough senses of humor. Tony was called "Hema" for all four years — long after the traumatic first months of his internship in which he single-handedly drained the hospital's blood supply.

Waldo might have cleaned up his act, but some problem children never did. Some of the worst to deal with were the lazy ones. We had a third-year who constantly hung her interns out to dry. She forced them to do procedures on their own that she should have guided them through and tried to do the least amount of work of any doctor I'd seen since the World's Worst Intern. I guess that made her the World's Worst Third-Year.

I hauled her into a conference room and yelled at her for a while, but it didn't make a lot of difference. The problem was, and still is in most residency programs, that there aren't good procedures for getting rid of that kind of person. You really have to screw up in a flamboyant way to wash out of a residency. The lazy ones — the undependable ones — the excuse-makers — the ones bad enough to make it hard on everyone they work with, but not bad enough to kill someone. They slide by. If you start to squeeze them, then the lawyers get involved so you're stuck with them. I also think that a lot of program directors have a vested interest in getting people through the four years in a nice, efficient way. It makes the residency program look good. In my twenty-five years of practice only a couple of people haven't made it through a residency. That's really a problem with the system.

Then there are the residents who want to do a good job but don't have the emotional equipment for it. I remember a resident who almost certainly had some sort of personality disorder. It was impossible for her to prioritize what she learned from a patient. You'd ask her for a patient's history and every tiny detail of everything she knew — and that was always a lot — came out in a shapeless mass of data delivered in monotone. As a diagnostician, she was highly thorough and yet nearly worthless. Every fact had the same weight. It was just as important where the patient had gone to high school as the fact that she'd been bleeding for thirty days. At some point in her recital I always had to rein her in.

"Okay. She seems ready to deliver. Let's focus on that and talk about her dog's name later."

That resident had to repeat her internship, something that seldom happens.

I saw another young intern come close to suicide because he simply couldn't handle the pressure. In the cafeteria one morning a chief was deep in discussion with one of his interns and it was clear from their expressions that the subject was serious. I thought that maybe the kid's mother had died. After they finished breakfast I asked the chief what was going on. He said that the intern had told him he was driving ninety miles per hour to work that morning hoping that he would crash. He was admitted to the hospital that day because of the suicidal tendencies, and he never came back to the program. He's succeeded notably in another profession, I'm happy to say, but he wasn't suited for medicine.

It's sad. I've seen a lot of kids get channeled into a medical career because of family expectations. Maybe a parent was a doctor or being a doctor was considered the pinnacle of professional success. Since childhood, these people were always going to be MDs. They went through their early lives with tunnel vision, straight through med school into a residency, and when they couldn't do the job they were devastated. That must be a frightening place to be and I felt lucky that I had come to my career late and with a taste of life on the outside.

The problem children and the misfits are always there, and every resident from interns on up gets to know who they are. But it's the chief who has to deal with them directly about their issues and who sees the human overview — sometimes maddening and sometimes poignant. The case load you give up as chief is replaced with such things. They can be unpleasant, but that's the burden of authority.

Since I wasn't called in unless the case was difficult or unusual, the cases that I did get in the fourth year were memorable. One started with a call I got at home one night from my second-year.

"I've got a patient here that you're going to have to help me evaluate. I've never seen anything like this."

"Okay. Tell me the story."

"Kevin, I'd rather just have you come in and hear it for yourself."

I trusted this doc, so I didn't push it and I went in. The story was worth waiting for. The patient was admitted in a lot of pain, was short of breath, had difficulty walking, and had a broom in her vagina. The sweeping part was sticking out between her legs along with a few feet of handle. She said that she had been cleaning house in the nude and was in her bathroom. There was a cobweb up in a corner of the ceiling, so she set the broom against the sink, put one foot on the toilet, the other on the sink and reached up with a dust rag to get the web. At the top of her reach she slipped, fell, and the broom handle went in her vagina.

I'm afraid to say that we didn't believe anything she told us. That wasn't simply because of the bizarre circumstances or the sexual aspects of a broom handle in the vagina. All that had an obvious effect, but the other part had to do with patients' stories in general. Patients lie. All the time. About important things that you would think no one would lie about. About obvious things that you would think no one would try to hide. When it concerns patient stories doctors are battle-hardened cynics. So we kept asking skeptical questions that were probably annoying or insulting, but we had to do our job. She stuck to her story.

We were able, very carefully, to get her up to radiology and onto an x-ray table and then waited to hear from the radiologist. When we did we started to believe the story. The broom had wounded her with traumatic force. It had entered her vagina, traveled over her bowel, around her liver, through her diaphragm, and pierced her lung. We knew that the liver hadn't been pierced because there wasn't enough blood. That could have been fatal. She was the luckiest unlucky person I ever met.

We took her into surgery, got the broom out, and then we had to remove all the splinters. It was a long surgery. I got to the hospital around 10:00 that night and finished up around 7:00 in the morning. There was a team of doctors, including a general surgeon, a vascular surgeon, a pulmonologist, and the OBs. Our part was very small because all we needed to do was close the vagina. That sort of cross-departmental team, by the way, is something that only a chief could assemble. There's nothing in the rules to keep a second-year OB from calling the vascular surgery service, but they're going to want to talk to your chief or an attending about something in their field. A second-year doesn't have the proper status and that's just the way it is. Most importantly for this case, the patient made a full recovery. I'll bet that she never cleaned in the nude again.

OBs are called upon more than most specialties to take sexual histories and it's awkward. It seems unnatural to ask such deeply personal questions no matter how long you've been doing it. The answers are sometimes so funny that it's hard to keep from laughing out loud.

"Are you sexually active?"

"No, I just kind of lie there."

And, speaking of lying, that tendency of the patient to avoid the truth is even stronger when there are sexual angles involved. A history taken by an intern sounds something like this:

"The patient is an eighteen-year-old who's never been pregnant. Her last period was three weeks ago. She's never had sex, but she's having abdominal pain and some bleeding."

A second-year will say, "I've got an eighteen-year-old who claims to be a virgin and is having some abdominal pain and bleeding and has a positive pregnancy test."

To be fair to the patient, they don't know what information the doctor really needs and so they'll lie about very important things that they think are unimportant. Their age, for example. That's a big factor in correct diagnosis for a doctor and a simple issue of vanity to a patient. Likewise, when an OB is trying to date a pregnancy the patient will try to place the conception when her boyfriend was home from the service and not when he was in Germany.

Eventually, experience teaches the doctor what questions to ask. I had been seeing our patient Isobel since I was an intern — through two unplanned births and a lot of interviews and second-guessing. She was using birth control pills but that didn't stop the pregnancies. We thought that she was missing doses somehow or might have had interference from other medications. By the time I was a chief, I was finally starting to learn what to ask and to learn the first commandment is Take Nothing For Granted. When I asked Isobel to describe exactly how she administered the birth control pills I finally figured out the problem. My first clue was when she said that they kept falling out.

"Isobel, are you putting the pills into your vagina?"

"They're for birth control," she said. "Where else would I put them?"

Of all the memories of my chief's year our winter retreat is front and center. To me, it's a symbol of my effort to make an impact as chief. The retreat still comes up in conversation with my St. Francis compatriots, so I guess the effort worked. On the other hand, becoming legendary is not always a good thing.

That issue of communication within the department still concerned me so I got the idea that if we chiefs couldn't change the way the residency program was structured then maybe we could change the way the people inside that structure worked together. A weekend retreat seemed the ideal solution. We'd spend two days together getting to know each other better, talking out problems, bonding — all the good stuff that retreats are supposed to do. The universal reaction to my idea was something along the lines of "Are you out of your mind?" Other good questions followed: "Who will staff the department for two days?" "Where could we all go for a weekend that we could even begin to afford?" "Do you seriously think that Gibbons is going to let us go on retreat?"

The staffing question was tough, but I thought that maybe we could talk some of the younger attendings into covering for us just for two days. They had been in our shoes not too long ago, remembered what it was like, and many of us were friends with them. Three agreed — good old Kenny "Don't Fuck Up" Gordon among them. Thanks to a complaining husband one of our residents wasn't going that gave us enough coverage to make the plan work.

One of our third-years came up with the perfect place. Her parents owned a vacation cabin in the White Mountains straddling the Vermont–New Hampshire border and were happy to let us use it. A cabin in the White Mountains during skiing season? Things were definitely taking shape.

The question about getting Gibbons's permission seemed the toughest. Taking a weekend off during the middle of the residency year was unheard of. He had invited me to his office and I sat across from him at his desk. He was always so elegant and well-spoken that, despite his friendliness, I felt intimidated. When I told him that I thought a retreat might improve the morale of the residents he was puzzled.

"What morale problems do we have? Are some of the residents dissatisfied?"

"I wouldn't say they're dissatisfied, but there are problems that need to be discussed. As for what the problems are, I'd rather not go into that. That's really between the residents."

He looked at me silently for a few seconds, and I thought that my last comment had blown it. Then he opened a desk drawer and pulled out a checkbook.

"Here's two hundred and fifty dollars. Have dinner on me Saturday night."

I couldn't believe it! That was when two hundred and fifty dollars could buy a pretty good meal for that many people. That was John Gibbons.

So on a Friday morning in February all the ob-gyn residents at St. Francis minus one piled into cars and headed to Vermont. There were no spouses or significant others invited. I felt guilty leaving Nancy with the kids, but it was a business meeting and at least I had been spending more time at home that year. (Lucy, the third-year whose husband threw a fit, ended up taking call on Saturday night all by herself. I wondered what that would do for their marital relations.) Twelve of us straggled up to the cabin in time to do some late afternoon skiing at the resort next door and end the day with food, drinks, and talk around an open fire. Things were working just the way I had hoped.

It should be noted here that I'm not a good skier, and at that point I had just learned, so I was even less skilled than I am now. I stuck to the easy slopes, the "greens," and there was supposed to be a very nice green run up at the top of the mountain. On Saturday I stayed around the cabin enjoying what I saw as our increasing camaraderie. By the time I headed for the mountain it was the middle of the afternoon.

"Will I have enough time to do that green trail?" I asked Ellen, whose parents owned the cabin.

"Oh, yeah! Just go up to the top and look for the green. It comes all the way down. It'll be your last run of the day and it'll be perfect."

I went up to the top of the mountain and looked around and all the trails were double black diamonds. Expert slopes. I finally went over to the ski lift operator to get some help.

"Somebody told me there was a green up here."

"Well," he said, "it's not a green; it's a blue. You can get to it by going down this double black diamond a little ways."

Oh, brother. I went over to the expert double black diamond and then had to slide down sitting on my skis a few hundred yards to the blue. I wasn't going very quickly butt-skiing, but the uncomfortable fantasy of accelerating out of control over a ledge kept playing out in my head. "Hartford Doctor Found At Bottom Of Cliff." I finally reached the blue run. It was all ice. I tried to ski, but I simply couldn't stop. I'd take off diagonally with a loud terrifying hiss like a fire hose as my skis slid across the trail into the woods. Crash. Up on the skis again. Hissssss. Crash. Hissssss. Crash. Good times.

It was starting to get dark, and I'd only made it about a quarter of the way down the mountain. When I looked back up I saw a whole gang of skiers watching me. So I waited for them to pass me and they kept waiting for me. Oh, hell. Hissssss. Crash. Hissssss. Crash. Finally, my audience took off down the run and passed me — all except for one woman. She came over to me and it turned out that they were the Ski Patrol. They were closing the mountain for the night; I was the last person up there.

She was giving me pointers and moral support and my thighs were screaming. I couldn't turn on that ice. Finally, she said, "I don't think we're ever going to get down the hill at this rate. I'm going to call the snowmobile."

Up it came. What an indignity. But it felt good to be moving straight down the slope with no detours into the woods. When we got to the bottom, though, there was no one there. Not a light in a window; not a car in the lot. All my friends had gone back to the cabin, and I had no ride. So I got my rubbery, aching legs moving and began to walk the mile back to the cabin in my ski boots through four feet of snow.

When I got there it was about 7:30, dark and biting cold, and as I went up the front walk lurching like Frankenstein I could see everyone inside — all eleven of my former friends — sitting around the table eating John Gibbons's dinner and having a fine time. The effort to create camaraderie was a clear success — except for the part about leaving your chief on the mountain. I pushed through the door and there was a roar of greetings.

"Kevin! Where have you been, man? We were wondering about you!"

I was testy but after chugging a hot cocoa and then digging a little more slowly into the food, I began to feel human again. We sat around the table late that night, talked and laughed about the hospital, aired a few grievances, discussed some problems, and enjoyed ourselves. The evening ended with the bestowing of nicknames. Each of us got named after one of the attending physicians we were supposed to resemble and for the rest of our residencies that's what we were called. I became Ron Czaja after the big, lumbering, unruffled doc who refused to be hurried. I like to think that it was given because of my reliable behavior in times of crisis and not because of the way I waddled around the cabin after my ordeal. Nobody really liked their nicknames. They were another example of the tough humor of medical people.

The retreat was a success though. We still talk about it, and especially about the story called (depending on who's telling it) "The Time You Got Lost On The Mountain" or "The Time You Left Me On The Mountain."

As my fourth year swept to a close, things seemed to move faster. The retreat was in February and in four months I was going to be out on my own. I was getting a taste of that already. Connecticut gives residents a medical license during their fourth year, so in the free time that I had as a chief I had already begun working at an urgent care office, a "Doc in The Box." I loved it, though I was treating patients for things far from my ob-gyn expertise, like flu, sprained backs, smashed thumbs. There were no life-threatening emergencies, and I was glad of that. It was a wonderful thing to be practicing free of the hospital. As grateful as I was to St. Francis and as much as I cared about the people there, I was ready to be gone. Senioritis. The goal for four years had been private practice and in a few weeks I would be there. "Where are you going in July?" was a constant question.

In a sense, the entire residency is a job interview, and I tuned into that fact late. I started actively looking for jobs in my fourth year, but I should have been doing that earlier — putting out feelers, asking the doctors I met in my electives about openings, writing letters. I had always felt too busy, but now I had to step it up and I was talking with attendings I knew both in Connecticut and Ohio.

Nancy and I wanted to stay in Hartford to build our first practice. We had grown fond of the place and the people, and the kids agreed. They had objected loudly about the move to Connecticut and now they objected loudly about a move back to Ohio. Four years is a long time to a young person and their roots were deep into Hartford.

Anthony Talisi was one of the Hartford ob-gyns who seemed interested in me. I liked him and he was good — good hands and good with patients. (His brother, also an OB, was just the opposite — clumsy and with the worst hands of any doctor I'd ever seen. He eventually cut off one of his thumbs in a chainsaw accident. Everyone who told that story followed up with, "It figures.") Their family had become folklore at the hospital. They were rumored to be Family with a capital F. The dad was supposed to be a capo in some crime family or other. Tony was the only Talisi who mattered to me, though, and he couldn't decide about making an offer. He told me that he was going to think about the hire and give me a call in a week. That call has become part of our own family folklore. Occasionally, thirty years later, Nancy or I will wonder out loud if this is the weekend that Tony Talisi will call.

But I had been talking to Steve Peters, the head guy at Ohio State, since the beginning of the year, and he was the one who finally made me the offer I couldn't refuse. The university was opening a suburban Family Planning office and I could design and run an office in the general Ob-Gyn division. I told Steve that I didn't want to be an academic. Publish or perish was not for me. I just wanted to practice medicine, and he said that that was fine with him. In a couple of years it turned out to be not so fine with the university, but that bump was down the road.

I would be working with three other doctors. I did med school at Ohio State with one of them. Then there was a woman in her sixties who was close to retirement but wanted to build an adolescent gynecology practice. The fourth person had a background like Gibbons. She had been a surgery resident then moved into ob-gyn. It was a good group of people and I liked the idea of coming in at the start of a practice. The office was so new that part of the designing that Steve mentioned would include drapes and furniture. It was the best offer I'd had and after Nancy and I talked it over that's where we decided to go. It had become clear to us that Columbus was the place.

The last big event of the fourth year was the Chief's Dinner. All the residents and attendings get together and, as with the Where's Waldo's dinner, the jokes have the gloves off. Tony, Craig, and I got roasted and we roasted some of the attendings right back. I got to play Alex Trebek in a game of St. Francis Jeopardy. "Name an attending who has been arrested by the fashion police." That sort of thing.

What I was waiting for all evening was Vic Fortin's legendary Chief's Dinner joke. For four years I had been hearing about the joke that he told every year, but no one ever repeated it. That was

Vic's. He was a funny guy anyway and often had residents, nurses, and patients laughing. Jokes weren't his style, though, so I was fascinated by the prospect.

With everyone in the room chanting his name, Vic stood up and told one that was ridiculously corny, politely obscene, and worth the wait. I will follow the St. Francis tradition and won't repeat it here. Simply imagine someone you love telling a joke that you love a lot less. Vic Fortin was telling it, and everyone but the attendings, who had it memorized, had been waiting a long time to hear it, so it was like an earthquake in there. We loved him, and we loved his silly joke, and the chiefs loved being at the end of our long trek at St. Francis.

The dinner was a fitting way to mark the end of the residency. No pomp and circumstance and a lot of laughs. Medical people aren't sentimental. One of the things that always struck me about the residency program was the way momentous events would rush past unacknowledged in the daily schedule. People were just too busy to make much ceremony. That summer I got to the end of a quest that Nancy and I had set out on so long ago. We had made it through four years of medical school, four years of a residency, and I was now a licensed doctor. But there was no graduation ceremony, no commemoration of that very big event. There were just handshakes, hugs, promises to stay in touch, and the changing of the residency year with a new crop of quivering interns following blood trails down the halls. It was exhilarating, sad, and over in a flash. A new part of the journey was about to begin.

That May, Nancy, the kids, and I went to Disney World to celebrate, reconnect, and wind down. It was ideal. We stood in line for rides, got sunburned, ate wonderfully unhealthy food, and relaxed in a way we hadn't been able to do for four years.

It felt good.

Chapter 10

Old College Try

In Which I Find Academic Medicine Is Not for Me

My first try at private practice started lonely and ended badly, but the two years in between were a hell of an education. When Nancy and I decided to come back to Ohio State, we assumed that it would be together, but financial realities decided otherwise. What had been a hot seller's market in Hartford a few years before turned cold by the summer after my residency. The house just wouldn't move, and we couldn't afford two mortgages. So I came back to Columbus alone and, once again, lived with my parents. Nancy stayed to show the house and in the dim, dark days of landline long-distance calls we ran up quite a phone bill.

So those first months were spent missing Nancy and the kids and getting used to the new practice. As Steve Peters had promised, it was a ground-up operation. My partners and I did indeed get to choose the drapes and furniture and decide on which offices we got. That was sort of fun, but I thought that it was a problem that we had the time to do it. After four years of an intense workload at St. Francis I suddenly had a lot of spare time. It was a huge change — from working a hundred-hour week and taking call every third night to taking call one night a week and every fourth weekend. The days were easy, too. I did a half-day at the OSU student health clinic, a half-day covering the residents as a teacher, one day in the hospital, and the other three days were office hours. When you start a practice, though, you don't begin with many patients, maybe three or four a day. So the smart thing to do is to schedule them together. It's more efficient and it makes you look like you have a big practice.

Vic Fortin had always been good with that kind of practical advice and now I was using it. He also told us that if we did schedule our patients together to make sure we had an office with a back door. One of his former residents had blocked out his skimpy patient list to get them all into the office at once. He was back in an exam room doing a cervical polypectomy on a patient when she let out a horrible scream and began to bleed. He couldn't get the bleeding stopped and had to call the emergency squad. In front of his entire practice, the EMTs came in and took the screaming, bleeding woman out the front door. It took the guy's practice, Vic told us, a long time to recover.

So I had a back door, a few patients, a lot of free time, and I didn't much care for it. It was institutional culture shock and it had to do with far more than just the easy schedule. There also was a deep difference in the way small, private St. Francis

Hospital and huge, academic Ohio State University Hospital did things. My first Thursday at OSU was an eye-opener. The four of us in the practice each had a day when we would go to the main hospital, take care of our laboring patients, and do all our surgeries. Mine was Thursday. I scheduled all my surgeries in the morning — three hysterectomies starting at 7:30. I thought I would get the surgeries done, do my charting and get home about 5:00. A perfect day.

I showed up at 7:00 a.m. and the OR coordinator told me that I wouldn't be able to start at 7:30. Moon Lee (kind of the second-in-command after Steve Peters) had to retrieve some eggs from a patient for an in-vitro procedure. The woman was ovulating, and the opportunity had to be taken. I understood emergencies. I'm in obstetrics.

Moon Lee did his egg retrieval, and then it turned out that he had two of them to do. So I got bumped again. I finally got started about 10:30 and got through at 12:30 p.m. I thought that I could get started on my second case about 1:00 and get more or less back on schedule. No. It took them two and a half hours to turn over the room. At St. Francis, an OR would be ready for the next patient in a half hour. At OSU that could be doubled or tripled.

That's because at an academic hospital you're teaching anesthesiologists, nurses, med students, young residents — everybody involved. In effect, you're scheduling a class as well as a surgical procedure, so everything's more complicated. And at St. Francis everyone was getting paid by the case. The motivation was to move through surgeries as efficiently as possible. Ohio State was civil service. They got paid by the hour and they didn't get any overtime. By 3:00 I still had two hysterectomies to do. Or so I thought.

The OR coordinator said, "Well, we're going to get started at 3:15, but we'll have to get some overtime approved first because everybody goes home at 3:30."

I said, "Wait a minute. You can't do emergency surgeries after 3:30?"

"Oh, yeah. We can do emergencies. That's why some of the staff stays. But it's really a skeleton crew."

Oh. Hmmm.

We did the second hysterectomy and then they told me that since it was so late the third patient had been put on the emergency list. As an elective surgery on a list of emergencies she would be a very low priority. Basically, she was out of luck.

I couldn't believe it. Everybody went home at 3:30 and my patient who was scheduled for noon gets put on a damned waiting list. She had been NPO (nil per os) — nothing by mouth — since midnight. No food and no water. I went to find her to see how she was doing and explain the situation and I discovered that she hadn't even had an IV. This was late afternoon and she had gone seventeen hours without food or water and not even an IV to give her some hydration. I was in a slow burn as I waited for the IV to come.

A nurse came up to me and said, "Your patient says she has a terrible headache."

"No shit she has a terrible headache! She hasn't had any food or water for about a day!"

The nurse ran off and then I felt even worse. It wasn't her fault. It was the system I was working in. I asked myself if I had made a mistake.

Finally, about 7:00 p.m. they told me that they were going to send my patient into surgery. Hallelujah. So I sat in the scrub room of the OR waiting and waiting and waiting. She didn't show up.

I called the OR people. "Where's my patient?"

"We sent transportation to get her and she should be there any minute."

"Well, can I go and get her?"

"Oh, no. You can't do that. That's against regulations. Transportation has to do it."

I guess I wasn't listening hard enough. I went up to her room. She wasn't there, and her room was next to the elevator. So was the OR. So I went back down there. The transportation guy came rolling her up from the direction of another hospital building. At that point I just wanted to get her into surgery, so I didn't even ask how he had enjoyed his trip. The hysterectomy, thank God, went well and I got home about 10:00.

After a few weeks of this kind of thing Nancy said to me, "You know, every Thursday when you get home your knuckles are white."

Bureaucracy. That's the university hospital. In that sort of civil service environment the person with the most power is the unit coordinator, the one who schedules the surgeries. Way down the pyramid are the doctors and nurses — far below the bureaucrats. There was another incident in those first few months that brought home to me the power of the bureaucracy.

Kevin Wilson was a doctor I had gone through med school with. He got out before I did and had been an attending at Ohio State for a few years. He had been one of the best students in the old days, and he had a great reputation now. It was a lot of fun to be reunited with him and to catch up on the friendship.

One Thursday at the hospital Kevin told me that he had been scheduled to do a laser biopsy when he was informed that his name wasn't on the approved laser list. Now, he had been doing laser surgery at OSU for about twelve years; he had been trained in it there as a resident and he had used it repeatedly as an attending. Then suddenly his name wasn't on the laser list and he couldn't do the surgery he had scheduled. He went to the guy who kept the list, a guy who had been working there ten years, and asked him what the hell was going on.

"Look," he told him, "It's me. You know me. This is obviously a mistake. We've done this procedure together dozens of times. Put me back on the list. I need to take care of this patient."

"I'm sorry. Rules are rules. I can't let you do the laser surgery because you're not on the laser list."

When Kevin told me all this I said, "Listen, I *am* on the approved laser list, so I'll proctor you."

So Kevin had to take me as a proctor, the person that he had taught the technique to six years before. I just stood there and watched him do it. He did a great job. He'd been well-trained.

That was typical of Ohio State. There were problems on other fronts, too. The business side of the new practice wasn't running smoothly.

First of all, one major shortcoming of medical education is that they don't train you in business. The closest they come these days is a little bit of work in insurance coding and billing, but they don't really teach you how to run your own shop.

Most people who come out of a residency join a group, so it's not essential to know your way around a spreadsheet. If you're interested, you can take some time to learn then. But if you want to work solo you've got to know what you're doing. You can't just hang out a shingle and start seeing patients. You've got to know accounting, marketing, tax law, Medicare and Social Security regulations, all sorts of things. A lot of doctors end up learning these things in the school of hard knocks. I had a terrific advantage over most of my colleagues because I had come out of business, yet I was still a babe in the woods when it came to running a medical office.

The practice at Ohio State that I joined was a fairly large collection of doctors. There were four of us in the general Ob-Gyn division, but there were a lot of people in other subspecialties — maternal fetal medicine, oncology, endocrine infertility. Thirty people altogether. It was all one corporation, so we had business meetings and at these meetings it was soon obvious to me that few of the doctors there had even a glimmer about what was going on or how the practice was doing. At one of these meetings we'd been reviewing accounts receivable and accounts payable on the quarterly report. One of my partners turned to me and said, "I don't know why you're saying that we're not doing so well. These income figures look great to me."

"Mike," I said, "When account numbers are shown in parentheses that means they are negative numbers. Our profit figure down here is in parentheses. It's a loss."

There were a lot of losses that first year. That's not unusual in a new practice, but that reality was aggravated for me by what I saw as an adversarial attitude by the university. From the haphazard way we were informed, I wasn't even sure that they *wanted* the doctors to understand the business side. My earlier contract negotiations got me thinking in that direction. There had been some stipulations in the contract that gave the hospital a lot of power and the resident very little.

It's not just balance sheets that doctors struggle with. We struggle with contracts, too. I did with the Ohio State contract, but I was lucky enough to have a brother who's a lawyer. My growing headache while suffering over the contract sent me to Tony. Tony made only a couple of changes making me wonder why I bothered, but two years later I realized how valuable they were. The contract stated that I wouldn't receive a bonus in the year I left the hospital. Tony changed that along with a clause that kept me from practicing within twenty-five miles of Ohio State after I left. The real effect of the lengthy, detailed, tightly woven contract — the real *bottom line* as it were — is that it made me feel like a potentially troublesome employee rather than a valued colleague.

While I was trying to find my feet in the new environment in Columbus, Nancy was dealing with the house and the family back in Hartford.

We had a realtor, of course, and she would let me know when we had a showing or an open house. So my main job was keeping the house presentable and that wasn't always easy. With the kids out of school things were hectic to say the least. They tried to be helpful, though, and we just did what we had to do. That was one of the important things we learned to do as a family as Kevin worked toward his medical license — how to set our minds on something and get it done. The incident that really stands out in my memory of the time was getting trapped in our bedroom and losing our dream buyer. Not in that order, actually.

It could get pretty loud in the house when all of the kids were home, and I would often go upstairs to the bedroom for important calls. I was up there one afternoon making some and when I tried to open the door the knob didn't work. It turned but nothing happened. The door wouldn't open, and I was stuck. I spent some time trying to play with the knob, but nothing worked. I pounded on the door and Tim, who was fourteen, came up and tried to help. Nothing worked, and so Tim walked down to the bottom of the hill where there was a fire station and in a little while I could hear sirens heading back up the hill and a huge fire truck parked out in front. As I was thinking of crawling under the bed, the phone rang and it was Kevin. He sounded upset and I said,

"Oh, my God, how did you hear about the fire truck so quickly?"

He said, "What?! Fire truck? Are you okay?"

When we both got calmed down it turned out that he had been calling to tell me that our buyer had backed out. The realtor had called him instead of me. All I wanted at that point was to save the bedroom door for the next buyer, so I was trying to tell the firefighters through the door to go easy on it. They got it open, but there was damage which one of our great neighbors, John O'Connor, fixed before the next showing. That was so kind of him, but I think he also just wanted to keep hearing the story.

With school approaching, Kevin and I finally decided to bite the bullet and pay for two mortgages. So he found a

house in Columbus and I got the place in Hartford emptied
out and the kids and I headed for Ohio. It was bittersweet to
look at that empty house, but it felt so good to accomplish
our dream. Kevin and I were done with his education and
ready to start the real deal.

I think, all in all, that I had it easier. We lucked out, though. The realtor finally came up with a buyer, and the day Nancy and the kids got to Columbus the closing papers for the Hartford house were in the mailbox. We're still in the house we found in Columbus.

One of my first deliveries at Ohio State was a woman who reached me at home, thought she was going into labor, and went into the hospital. I called in some orders and told them to call me when she was eight centimeters and I'd come down. She progressed normally, and I drove down, gowned up, and went to the delivery room.

The nurse said, "Wow! Isn't it wonderful when patients go into normal labor at term and just have their baby with no problems?"

I was at a loss, but finally said, "I hope that's what *all* my patients are going to do!"

That gives you an idea of the environment at an academic hospital. Ohio State is a tertiary care center, at the top of a pyramid of local and regional hospitals. We got referrals for very complicated, high-risk patients from all over the state. Pre-term, diabetic, and hypertensive patients are the norm.

On my first night supervising the residents I got nervous just looking at the patient board. There were lots of extremely sick patients. We had one woman sent from Marietta whose doctor wanted to know if she had preeclampsia. Back in those days we diagnosed preeclampsia from high blood pressure, protein in the urine, and whether they had complications such as seizures.

This patient was born with a seizure disorder, had chronic renal failure so she was spilling protein into her urine, and had had hypertension since she was twelve years old. When it came to diagnosing preeclampsia I wondered how we were supposed to do that, but that was OSU.

I went in for my first C-section and the intern started telling me about the patient next door who was having a ten-pound breech baby and it was her first child.

I said, "I'm not covering *that*, that's for the maternal fetal medicine specialist. Who's in there right now?"

"The other intern."

"I mean who is covering that patient? That can't be the intern."

"Well, we called Yuri Sirken and he said, 'Kevin is there. I know Kevin and he can handle it.'"

Yuri Sirken was the MFM specialist and seemed to have far more faith in my abilities than I did. I sure didn't feel like I could handle it. I was upset and said to the intern, "I'm not going to do a ten-pound breech first birth without a C-section. We need to section that patient."

"No," the intern said, "We're going to do a vaginal delivery because the baby has a lethal anomaly. It's not going to survive."

Then I understood. It was another of the difficult cases I had been seeing so often. The way the case had been communicated to me was a problem, though — another small warning sign to me about where I was and what I was doing.

All the difficult and high-risk cases I was seeing were going to be important in another way. After the second year as an attending I needed to go before the medical board for certification. It's sort of like getting an advanced degree — not essential to practice, but an additional professional accomplishment. A lot of universities insist that their attending physicians get board certified and Ohio State was one of those universities. During the first year as an attending, doctors applying for certification are required to collect their most challenging cases for presentation to the board after their second year. I certainly wasn't going to have a problem with finding challenging cases, but I wanted to make sure that I knew everything there was to know about them.

One of the difficult cases was an elderly woman who had complete procedentia; her uterus and vagina were outside the body. She no longer had any use for her vagina and wanted it closed up, but everything on the outside had to go back in and that's hard to do. I dug through the literature and found a surgical technique for this situation that had been done by Gunther

Riefenstuhl in Germany during World War II. It was an old technique, and the medical ethics of that period in Germany was questionable, but it looked good on the page, and it turned out to be an excellent surgery. The organs are circumscribed by the scalpel and purse-string sutured; they collapse and then can go back up and into the body.

The guy assisting me, John Thompson, kept saying, "This is so cool!"

And it was. Doctors can be such nerds about a good technique and this was one. John also asked me how many of these procedures I had done. I hated to tell him it was the first. I was almost reading out of the book as we did it. I think I did have it available in the scrub room.

John, who was a third-year resident, also assisted me on a case that I have never encountered since — a ruptured uterus in a first-time mother with no surgical history. This young woman had given birth easily with a fast labor but had lacerated her cervix. It split. It's not clear why that happens, and it happens very rarely, but here it was. Most of the time when that happens the split only goes a little way. Not hers. We kept stitching and stitching until we realized that we'd have to go all the way up to the top of the uterus, inside the abdomen. It was as rare a case as you could find. We had to open her up and repair the uterus from above. It took hours and I was sweating literally and figuratively. John and I got things under control, and the patient simply went home a week or two later than she expected. The seriousness of the laceration wasn't anybody's fault. It was just the kind of bad luck that sometimes happens, but I still felt responsible. Most doctors do. And I thought I would be raked over the coals about the case during my board orals.

The boards! They loomed large and intimidating during my first year of practice.

Fred Zimmerman, the guy — himself intimidating — who had put the clock on his desk during my residency interview, led a preparation course for the boards and I was happy to take it. Zimmerman was a board examiner himself, but when he was working on your side that intimidating demeanor was reassuring. We took classes during the day, then in the evening we'd sit around and have an oral exam with Fred moderating. I got two things out of the class. It made me ready for the oral boards and it also showed me how unprepared some people are. There were doctors there who were not going to pass. I felt sorry for them, but it was also reassuring somehow. Maybe, I thought, all it takes to get through the ordeal is solid preparation.

They gave the boards in a hotel in Chicago, the Francis Drake. I checked in and headed up in the elevator to my room. Mingling or sightseeing had no appeal; I just wanted to study until bedtime. My anxiety level was already redlining, and I wasn't sure I'd be able to sleep. Unfortunately, I got there just as the day's exams were over and my elevator stopped on that floor. It was like the elevators that take you to the floor where the fire is. All these blathering, punch-drunk examinees were standing in the foyer obsessing to each other about what had just happened to them. It was a cacophony of anxiety.

Then they staggered into my elevator and continued the self-flagellation. It was disheartening. I lay awake for a long time, but finally did get to sleep. The exam turned out to be easier than I had expected — tough, but manageable. They didn't ask any questions about those tough cases I was so worried about. I've realized since that the examiners have their own agenda of issues and problems that they want to cover and if they find something in the histories you've submitted that lets them do that then you'll hear about your cases. They don't rummage through your cases to find things to nail you about. Thank God. Thank Fred Zimmerman, too. Of course his residents would say that's redundant.

After two years at OSU I was board certified, had received a great education in high-risk ob-gyn and had become deeply interested in teaching. In so many ways I couldn't have asked for a better place to start my career, but I was realizing that I wanted something different — more opportunity to work with normal pregnancies in a less stressful setting. I don't think I was a Pollyanna trying to avoid the tough cases, but sometimes it seemed like all we *got* were the tough cases. I kept remembering that nurse who seemed awestruck at a normal full-term pregnancy and remembered, too, that my love for the field in medical school came from helping to bring patients the joy of a healthy birth. Then I had a fateful meeting with Steve Peters and my mind got made up for me.

When I came to OSU I had told Steve that even though I would be at an academic hospital, I wasn't interested in writing academic papers. Steve said that would be no problem. That all changed a couple weeks before Christmas. Steve asked me to stop by his office to talk about his textbook on ob-gyn, which was being edited for a new edition. Steve's book was so influential that doctors around the country referred to it simply as "Peters."

"Kevin, I want you to contribute a couple of chapters, one on clinical practice and one on menopausal medicine."

The first topic reflected my interest in practical ob-gyn, the sort of deep practical knowledge that I'd seen in Vic Fortin among others. Steve's awareness of my interest was flattering, but I still didn't want to write, even about that. And the second topic was a bit of a sore point. Menopausal gynecology was seen as a field of the future — to Steve and a lot of other doctors as well. As the baby boomers aged there would be more call for menopausal treatment. So Steve had enrolled me in a professional society of menopause medicine and had felt that that should be a focus of mine. I just wasn't interested, so we had already had that little tug-of-war and I had lost. Now he was telling me to write about it. On the way back down from Steve's office everything had changed. The hospital looked different to me. I knew I was gone; it wasn't my place any longer.

The next day I made a call to Connecticut and talked to Ron Czaja about coming back to Hartford. He and his partner Ron Gefeller had an opening and were enthusiastic about me coming back. When I brought it up at home, though, I got educated in a hurry. The kids hated the idea and hated it loudly. Since they hadn't wanted to come back to Ohio, I assumed that they would jump at the chance of going back again to see their friends. Dumb dad. I should have been more tuned in to their situations. They had been here for two years and that's a very long time to a young person.

While I was trying to sort all this out, we took a skiing trip to Colorado and one afternoon I got a call from Don Turner, my old boss and mentor back in Columbus, about an ob-gyn practice that was up for sale. A doctor in suburban Columbus wanted to move to Florida and the deal would include his office, his staff, and his patients. It was perfect for me, Nancy, and the kids and I jumped at it. It was hard to call Ron Czaja to tell him I wouldn't be coming after all, but I couldn't make any other choice.

There were still some loose ends to tie up at Ohio State, though, and the biggest of them was the amount of money that I still owed for my malpractice insurance. OSU had been paying for the insurance as part of my salary, but the coverage had to be continued in case a former patient sued me. The amount of that continued coverage, called a "tail," wasn't huge, because I'd been in practice only eighteen months. It was still around twenty thousand dollars, though, and Nancy and I didn't have that kind of money.

So I called Steve Sedlak, my old boss at the insurance company, and asked him if there was any work I could do down there. He told me that there was. I could modernize the actuarial programs that I had coded way back in '73 and '74. They were in COBAL and the company was switching to BASIC. So I was all set. Almost. Steve told me to come in on Monday and he'd have the stuff ready for me in his office. But the next day he called me.

"I made a big mistake."

"You don't need the work after all?"

"Oh, we need the work, but apparently I can't hire people without going through HR. So come down, talk to those guys and then you can start working."

So I went down to HR and they immediately started talking about my actuarial exams. I said, "I'm not *doing* actuarial work. I'm just doing computer programming. Part-time at night."

"But," they said, "Since you've had five actuarial exams you're going to need an office and a secretary, and you need to work at pay level three."

"Wait a minute," I said, "Steve's going to pay me ten dollars an hour to work at night programming. That's it. I'm not going to be an actuary."

So they huddled and decided that I didn't need a secretary or a particular pay grade, but I had to have an office. Bureaucracy again! Makes me crazy.

When Steve got the verdict he said, "I've got a hallway between two of the offices in my section. We'll just put a door on it and there's your office."

The hallway had been for window access, so I now had an office with a window — a long, narrow office. And I had my name on the door. I'd come in at night, drop off my printouts, and pick up my new work. I'd spend only three or four minutes in the office. After a few weeks of this I was told that I was becoming a legend. There was a mysterious doctor who worked only at night! Nobody ever saw him, but his work would disappear and the next morning the completed papers would show up on his desk. I guess I did sound like a campfire story: "The Ghost Doctor: Ob-Gyn by Day, Programmer by Night."

The other big loose end was negotiating with Steve Peters about my departure and it was uncomfortable. The meeting was in his office and there were only three of us — Steve, me, and an OSU accountant. We had to wade through a lot of dry details and the accountant was doing a lot of the talking, which is seldom a good thing. I had tried to explain as diplomatically as I could the reasons for leaving and what I planned to do next. When I described the new practice Steve perked up.

"It's in Westerville? Kevin, you can't practice in Westerville. We have a non-compete clause in our contract that keeps you from practicing within twenty-five miles of the hospital."

Silently singing Tony's praises I said, "No, Steve. We took that out."

He couldn't believe it and the accountant loudly rustled through my contract. After a couple very long minutes he surfaced and said, "He's right, Dr. Peters. Page 6."

A short time later I informed them how to get my yearly bonus to me.

"Kevin, the university doesn't pay a bonus in the last year of employment."

"Actually, we changed that, too."

The rustling started again. Two minutes later the accountant said, "Yeah. Page 6."

The meeting ended soon after. Steve was annoyed, the accountant was looking over his glasses at me like a peeved librarian, and I wanted to get out of there. No one wanted to reference Page 6 again.

I hated making Steve Peters angry. I admired the guy a lot. But what was also true was that as I drove out of the parking garage I felt better than I had felt in a long time. I was going to be my own boss. I was going to minimize the bureaucratic foolishness (no doctor can ever get rid of all of it). I was going to have a stable group of patients, and I could be their doctor over the long term. It was a terrific feeling that was going to get even better.

Almost Perfect

In Which I Try My Hand at Solo Practice

B ill Schmidt was a smart businessman and a genuine entrepreneur. He had a good-looking suburban office, a lot of patients, was an attending at three hospitals, and stayed on top of every new technology that came along. I admired all that, but we were about as different as two people could be. Bill was a flashy, supremely confident doctor with shining silver hair, a deep tan, and a gold chain around his neck. When he first showed me through his office I couldn't get over the huge photograph of his yacht that hung in the hallway outside the examination rooms. I wondered how his patients looked at that. With admiration? Awe? Envy? Did any of them think "My hysterectomy paid for *that*?"

Two of the new technologies that Bill adopted early were laser and laparoscopic surgery, and he even designed a course for teaching laparoscopy that was cheap, effective, and lucrative. He got the husband of one of his nurses to knock together a black, wooden box that had a rubber diaphragm on one side. Bill would make an incision in it, insert the laparoscope and remove a foam gall bladder for his class of general surgeons. The classes had a couple of hundred people in them, took a few hours each day for a week, and cost a thousand dollars per student. Those are encouraging numbers.

After I met Bill I told Don Turner, "This guy's a wheeler-dealer; I'm not like him at all. The patients won't know what to make of me."

"You don't have to be like him," Don said. "The patients probably aren't. Anyway, he'll be gone."

So we pulled the trigger. I bought the practice and arranged to pay Bill out of my profits while Don bought the office condo and leased it back to me. I kept all of Bill's staff, and the plan was that during the first six months he would work half the time, and I would work the other half and get introduced to the patients. The goal was a seamless transition. So much for goals. A couple of weeks after we closed the sale, Bill took off for Florida on his yacht, but before he left he played a prank that gave me a little insight into what our relationship would be like.

Bill was considering a fancy new ultrasound machine for the practice and he asked me to check it out. The salesman rolled the unit into an examination room, and Bill brought in a patient I had not met (which, at that point, described most of them) and then left. Amy was cooperative, but there was a strange reticence that I couldn't quite get a handle on. No matter; I was new to her. The machine was amazing — powerful and sensitive, with a better visual display than I'd ever seen. It was *what* I was seeing on that screen that was the problem. There were images of two uteruses. No matter how I tried to adjust the image there were still two uteruses. I thought that Vic Fortin had taught me well, but I began to think that maybe this machine was too much for me. I glanced up to clear my vision and saw the patient with the beginnings of a grin.

I said, "Amy, do you have two uteruses?"

She said, "Yeah, but Dr. Schmidt told me not to tell you."

That was a good example of a doctor not really seeing. I was sure the problem was with the machine or the way I was using it. Amy had two uteruses (uteri, to be proper), two cervixes, two vaginas. When an embryo develops, the sides of the uterus come together and the septum, the dividing wall between the sides, is eventually lost. If the process gets interrupted, though, the baby can end up with some of the reproductive organs doubled. It's very rare, but I had seen it before and had read about it in the literature. I was annoyed with myself for not seeing what was in front of me but pleased I had passed Bill's little test. I was less pleased with Bill. The whole episode seemed petty or juvenile. I wasn't sure exactly what to make of it, but it made me uncomfortable. It was a significant warning sign.

Then Bill was gone. He set course for Florida and it was quite a cruise. He traveled from Cleveland across Lake Erie, through the locks of the Erie Canal, into the Mohawk River, through Hudson's Bay into Chesapeake Bay and finally down the Inland Waterway to Sanibel Island. The trip took six weeks at the start of the transition time when the goal was to introduce me to my new practice. So I just introduced myself and was basically full-time from the start.

Being sans Bill turned out to be fine with me, though. I couldn't believe how much I loved solo practice. The ten years after I left Ohio State were the best of my entire career. That staff was great, I liked the patients, I was my own boss, and the whole situation had the kind of family feeling that I had been waiting for since I decided on ob-gyn. There were no business meetings, either. Driving to work in the morning I'd enjoy every minute just knowing that I was going there.

Before going solo, I had worried that taking call by myself 24/7 could be burdensome. It wasn't at all. My case load was smaller because I *was* solo — generally twenty pregnancies a month. About half of those ended up being night deliveries, so that meant one case every third night. Compared to my previous schedules that was cake. OBs get their schedule interrupted a lot, anyway. I'd get called out of the office for a delivery and be traveling around town in the middle of the day. Wonderful. Routine was at a minimum; it was freeing. And because I was solo I knew all the patients. In the OSU group, three-quarters of the patients were someone else's, so they were strangers. Knowing the patients really contributed to that family feeling and, more importantly, made me a much better doctor. That was the period when I began to feel that my experience was starting to sharpen my instincts — when I had flashes of becoming the doctor I wanted to be. Debbie Campbell comes to mind.

Broadly speaking, you can divide patients into two groups: the stoics and the alarmists. The stoics will bear just about anything in the way of pain or inconvenience and the alarmists will overreact for the smallest reason. It's not that one type is a good patient and one type is bad. Stoics can put themselves in grave danger by ignoring their symptoms, and alarmists, like paranoids, are sometimes right to be alarmed. Through the constant complaints of the alarmist, a doctor can sometimes catch something early.

Debbie was definitely a stoic. A century or so earlier, she could have been one of those women traveling West with the wagon trains with never a peep of complaint out of her. She was one of my Ohio State patients who had followed me into the solo practice. So I had gotten to know her, and when her husband called me a couple of days after Debbie had given birth to their first child I was uneasy. He said that she had come down with a bad cold and they were wondering how cold medications could affect her nursing of the baby. Knowing Debbie and her tendency to minimize, I knew more might be going on for her to have Don call me. I asked Don if I could speak to her. The moment Debbie began to talk I knew that we had a big problem. Her lungs were gurgling with every word. I said, "Debbie, you don't have a cold.

There's something more going on. You need to get to an emergency room."

By the time the squad got her there she was in heart failure — cardiomyopathy. There was so much fluid in her lungs that she could barely speak. It was a close call, but like I said Debbie is wagon-train tough and she recovered. Catching that problem by hearing her voice on the phone encouraged me. Maybe I was starting to get it.

Then about a year later, Debbie got in touch with me and told me she wanted to have another baby! I wasn't enthusiastic and told her that I was going to have to do some research. Peripartum cardiomyopathy is rare, and I didn't know if there were that many women who had had a baby after suffering from it. The figures were sobering. The risk of her dying in the next pregnancy was fifty percent. The risk of having heart failure again was eighty percent. Pioneer woman, though, thought those were acceptable odds.

"I don't want my daughter to be an only child," she said.

"That's better than being an orphan," I replied.

It was no use warning her, though; Debbie had her mind made up. So she got pregnant and I had her seeing a cardiologist every week. At thirty-four weeks I was thinking we'd better pull the trigger here and just deliver her or she's going to go into heart failure." But Debbie told me that she didn't want to go early and felt great.

The cardiologist called me on a Friday morning and said, "I just saw Debbie and she looks fantastic. She's got no symptoms and I think she can go another week."

I told him okay. Then four hours later I got a call from Debbie.

"Dr. Kington, I just don't feel right."

"Go on into the hospital and I'll meet you there."

As I was getting ready to leave for St. Ann's I got a call from an angry nurse.

"Dr. Kington you had no business sending that patient here! You should have sent her down to Ohio State to the heart transplant service. She's in heart failure and we're going to have to put in an A Line and there's no one here who knows how to do it except for Frank and ..."

"Calm down," I said. "Tell Frank to put in the A Line and I'll transfer her over to the heart transplant service." (An A Line is an arterial IV to measure oxygen and pressure.)

I wasn't that calm myself, but I'm usually able to hide that fact. So we went down to OSU in the middle of the night, went into the heart transplant room, put in a Swan-Ganz catheter, did her C-section, and tied her tubes. She wasn't going to get another chance to kill herself. I told her husband Dan,

"Your kid's not going to be an only child, but from now on you guys can adopt."

She was admitted to the cardiac care unit and intubated. Debbie was in sad shape and I didn't think that she would live.

Her ejection fraction — the measure of how efficiently her heart was pumping — was at twenty percent.

The next day when I did rounds on her she was starting to look pretty good and I let a little hope seep into my heart. But when I rounded on her the third day her bed was made. I knew what that meant. Why didn't they call me to tell me she had died? I liked Debbie a lot and it hit me hard. I found a nurse and asked, "Has Debbie died?"

"Oh, no," she said. "She was discharged this morning. She was feeling good, so she wanted to go home."

I was poleaxed. I could not believe it. Then I thought about who it was, and I believed it. Home from the cardiac care unit after two days! I thought I'd better give her a call the next day to see how she was doing and there was no answer. I was worried and left a message.

Debbie called back in a couple of hours and said, "Sorry I missed your call. I was out at the mall with the kids."

"At the mall? Holy God! Aren't you on oxygen?"

"Oh, yeah. I had to wheel the oxygen along with the stroller, but we did fine."

Her condition was related solely to pregnancy, so her heart's been fine ever since. Debbie is the most stoic of the stoics I've treated. I've wondered how things might have turned out if I hadn't asked Don to speak to her that day. But I did ask.

The alarmists outnumber the stoics by far. Some are just worriers and not without reason. One of the clinic patients of a St.

Ann's attending had had a ruptured uterus in a previous pregnancy and was sure that the same thing was happening. She was thirty-four weeks and was in terrible pain — screaming and thrashing. We couldn't tell if her uterus was rupturing, so I brought down the ultrasound and got her to hold still long enough to get a good image. I didn't see a rupture, but I did see a huge bladder. The division between it and the uterus was paper thin. I couldn't see if there was any uterine wall there so the bladder might have been covering a rupture. Her attending and I made an incision and did a laparoscopy and her uterus was perfect, but there was that huge, distended bladder. We emptied it and the pain was gone. She had convinced herself that she was rupturing, held in her urine, and the more that accumulated the more sure she was of the rupture. She probably had post-traumatic stress from that first episode.

A lot of patients, for one reason or another, are trying to convince their doctors that they're sicker than they are. Some of them, like the woman who just had to pee, are worriers. Some have ulterior motives. The two most common are pregnancy fatigue and drugs. Patients can simply get tired of being pregnant — the back pain, the kicking, the lack of energy, and physical limitations that come from carrying a baby. They want to be delivered, and if they can manipulate their physician into doing a C-section, they will.

I had one patient who insisted that she had preeclampsia and was experiencing seizures. When I went to her room to examine her, she was frantically waving her arms in front of her and saying that she had gone blind. That can be a symptom of preeclampsia, but I was skeptical. There seemed to be too much acting and too little real emotion. When I bent down to examine her I made a quick movement across her eyes with my hand and she flinched.

"Well, it looks like your vision has returned."

"Just now," she said. "It just now came back!"

She only wanted to get that baby out of there, but there are plenty of patients who fake terrible pain in an effort to get drugs. There are strong pain meds out there that are critically important in the treatment of those who really need them, but their abuse has become a big problem for doctors.

I never had many private patients who tried to trick me into giving them drugs. That's the upside of knowing your patients and being, in a sense, part of their extended family. There's a downside, though, and I was beginning to see how it affected my ambition to teach. If I wanted to pursue teaching I would need the kind of high-risk patients that I saw at Ohio State. Normal pregnancies with no complications are fine things for everyone involved, but there's nothing about them that an attending can use to teach a resident. Teaching meant too much to me to leave it behind, so I began to work two nights a week in the clinic of Grant Hospital in downtown Columbus. The difficult cases I saw in the clinic were a perfect balance with the normal pregnancies that made up most of my own practice.

Grant could be a wild place. Since it was right downtown, it was far more exciting than a sleepy suburban hospital. We had shooting victims, drug overdoses, and gang members eying each other in the waiting areas. And we had plenty of teachable ob-gyn cases.

On my first night there we got a call from Children's Hospital a few miles away. They had a pregnant woman in her thirty-second week there who had walked in to their clinic and was hemorrhaging. Patients in crisis don't always think clearly. She figured that a children's hospital was a good place to deliver a child, but didn't consider that she, the patient, was not one herself. The guy I talked to from Children's was a pediatrician, and he was pretty upset.

When we got her to Grant and diagnosed her, I couldn't understand why she was even in Columbus in the first place. She had a placenta previa. Her placenta was in front of the baby so that when she labored and the cervix dilated, she would hemorrhage. The placenta is in the way and the baby can't get out. That's what was starting to happen to her. It's such a potentially dangerous condition that when a patient has a placenta previa she needs to stay close to her doctor and her hospital. But Mary Lou had come up from West Virginia to visit her sister. She had no doubt ignored her doctors and it could have cost her her life.

She came wheeling in to the delivery room on a cart and had one of the bad signs of a pregnancy — blood between her toes. The only way to address a placenta previa is with a C-section so that's what we did. She had been bleeding a lot, but we worked quickly and she avoided DIC. She and her new son went home in a couple of days.

Another of those early Grant cases showed me how educational luck can be. Any doctor knows that disaster is a great teacher, but the opposite can be true as well. This patient went into pre-term labor and it was a face presentation. In a normal delivery the brow of the baby comes out first. When the face presents first the head is at an odd angle and the baby's forehead can get hung up on the mother's pubic bone. The nurse called me that night and told me that we had a face presentation and need to section the patient stat.

I went running down there, and I checked the patient to see how far dilated she was. When I put my hand in, the baby started sucking my finger and as I withdrew my hand she was sucking so hard that I delivered her. That's known as a modified Ritgen Maneuver and I learned it at that moment by the pure chance of finding a baby with a great sucking reflex. It saved the mom a C-section.

Some crazy things happened in the clinic. It fit with my sense of a hospital at night as being a strangely different world. One winter night I had delivered a young mother and stopped by her room where her family was gathered happily. Well, almost everyone was happy. Apparently there was still some question about the paternity of the little girl and two young men were there, each of whom knew that he was the father. They began to argue, and the argument moved out into the hall. Insults turned to shoves, and a nurse called security. The guys had their fists up when a big, red-faced security guard burst through the lobby doors, rushed over to them, pulled a canister out of his belt, and maced himself right in the face. He went down on his knees with a howl and after a beat of astounded silence, everyone else, including the two combatants, was howling, too — with laughter. The guys left quietly, possibly to argue again, but that night they were through. It was the most effective crowd control I've ever seen. We got the guard into an examination room, irrigated his eyes, and twenty minutes later he slinked away.

There was so much to like about my solo practice that I could have stayed there forever, but beneath the surface the foundations were eroding. Bill Schmidt and I never really got along. We never really trusted or liked each other. More importantly, we had fundamentally different views of our business arrangement. The original deal had been that whenever the practice was profitable Bill would get half the proceeds. After my experience in the group practice at Ohio State, I doubted that the practice would be profitable for a long time. Bill thought it would be profitable immediately. It turned out that the reason for our different views was that we had different definitions of profit.

The profits in the group practice had been spotty, and the same was true after going solo. We ran deficits for a few months, had a profitable period, then went back into the red. Between equipment, staff, and office, the practice had a whole lot of debt (that ultrasound machine was a backbreaker) and I thought that the debt needed to be paid down before we could call ourselves profitable. Bill, on the other hand, saw cash flow as profit, so if there was a spare dollar in the till at the end of a month he wanted fifty cents of it. We argued over that for years as I paid him. He always wanted more.

Eventually Bill's demands became threats and the threats became a lawsuit. I couldn't pay what Bill wanted and I had to declare bankruptcy. That was traumatic, both because the practice had to close and because I didn't like walking away from my debts. My dad had spent his entire career with a finance company, after all, and I didn't like thinking what he would say. I had no choice, though. I reached out to colleagues and was able to find a place in a friend's practice that would allow me to treat my patients, lick my wounds, and figure out what to do next. It was a tough time for me personally and professionally, but it led to the most rewarding medicine I ever practiced.

Chapter 12

Transitions

In Which I Find the Perfect Fit

George Busonik was my soft place to fall. I had known him since med school and he was the perfect guy to start the healing process after the disaster with Bill Schmidt. We had cross-covered for each other for years, and now he gave me the opportunity to work out of his office while keeping a separate practice. Except for the cramped quarters, it was a good situation. Careful, deliberate, and kind, George was beloved by his patients, and I wasn't far behind them. If a patient had an appointment, though, she knew to call ahead. Careful and deliberate, in George's case, resulted in slow. His nurses fielded calls all day from scheduled patients.

"How far behind is George?"

"An hour right now. You're at 3:00? Better make it 4:30."

George was as thorough as any doctor I've known and answered every question and addressed every concern at length. He never left the examination room until his patient decided they were done. Those were fortunate patients. The downside was obvious in the number of folks sitting in the waiting room at night. George was signed up for the 5:00 to 7:00 evening shift at St. Ann's, and then came back to the office. Often he was there until 10:00.

Doctors have different styles. George is a novel, and I'm more of a short story. I try to answer my patient's questions fully and think I'm a careful doctor, but I'm not much for small talk. I'm not going to know what church you go to or that pancakes are your favorite breakfast food. I defer to my inner surgeon; I like action. It's not that quick and decisive is better than slow and deliberate or the other way around. You can drive off the road on either side. Deliberate can be a problem in an emergency and quick is always in danger of becoming sloppy. The saving grace of any good doctor is always self-criticism. That's another way of seeing what's in front of you. Most of the time what you're seeing is your case, but sometimes what you're seeing is you.

A case early in my time at George's is a good example of that tendency of mine to act quickly. I was in the office examining a patient with a late-term pregnancy when the baby's heartbeat dropped into the 70s — very low. There are various reasons why that happens, but it's always a threat to the life of the baby and if it goes on for more than five minutes you need to do a C-section. Vital signs can fluctuate, though, so I waited for about ninety seconds then did another reading. Same thing. I didn't have the equipment at the office to do a section, but we were right down the street from St. Ann's, so I got on the phone and called a nurse.

"I've got a tones-down multip at thirty-five weeks and I'm bringing her over for a stat C-section. Get the room ready."

"Tones down" told the nurse about the slow vital signs of the baby and because this patient had given birth before, she was a "multip," meaning with multiple pregnancies. That's important to know because previous deliveries make a major difference in the length of the labor and ease of delivery.

I was on red alert. It would have taken crucial minutes to wait for the squad just so they could simply roll her down the street. So we bundled into my car, I floored it, and we roared off, ran through a gas station to avoid a red light, and slalomed through the parking lot up to the ER. Out of the corner of my eye I could see the mom bracing against the dashboard and door. Everybody was gowned up and ready for us at the hospital. We ran her back to the delivery room and listened to the heartbeat and it was 140. The kid was fine. I was embarrassed, but not much. That's me. I'd rather have a wild ride and be wrong than play it safe and regret it. Another doctor might have waited longer. Maybe George would have. That's okay, too.

Because we had far less space at George's than at the old practice, my staff didn't like the new arrangement as much as I did. Jan, my nurse, had a stool at a counter; my receptionist worked out front with George's receptionist, and I had some examination rooms at the back of George's building. Jan wasn't fond of sitting on that stool, and I made a big mistake with her when we moved over from the old building. I chose to make the move between Christmas and New Year's to keep from disrupting our patients' schedules. It did, but it disrupted our own and Jan has a big family. A good staff will forgive your dumb ideas, though, and I had a good one.

There was a big benefit in working out of someone else's office; the office manager didn't report to me and I had no responsibilities in running the place. That freed me to do more clinic work, both downtown at Grant and at St. Ann's. The question I needed to begin asking myself was whether I needed more work.

As much as I enjoyed my calling, I had been ignoring a darker side to my work life for years — I'd say ever since I began my solo practice. Workaholism is a wry term, and the wryness diminishes the seriousness of what it describes. Some people even use it as a badge of honor, but the problems it creates are toxic. I was damaging my marriage and my health. Nancy was left running the household for long periods and when I was around I was constantly tired and not much help.

Unfair and unhealthy is a bad combination for a marriage. This was the period in which our kids were in middle school through high school. All the turmoil of adolescent life was roiling the Kington household, and I was gone for a lot of it. Sometimes I've asked myself if that was on purpose. I honestly can't answer that. I hope not. We truly did need the money. All those kids were headed for college and declaring bankruptcy was hard on the credit rating.

I was lucky, as always, to have Nancy as a partner. That's been clear so many times during my life and no more so than at that point when the solo practice fell apart and I went to George's. Nancy saw it this way.

> As I look back at that time, I can see the problem. But at the time it just seemed normal. Kevin has always worked hard. My sister used to say that if you gave Kevin a day he could come up with a job. We both were working hard. We had a partnership, and when he wasn't around I did what had to be done. In hindsight, I wish he had been there more, but that's what a doctor's life is like. I'm glad it changed, though.

I'm glad it changed, too, but it took a while. I always knew that I had a tendency to overwork. I like the intensity of focusing on a task and getting it accomplished. As I've said, any good doctor needs a touch of Obsessive-Compulsive Disorder. Too much leisure time drives me crazy. My years at St. Francis deepened that tendency. When I came back to Columbus to start the Ohio State practice, I found the spare time compared to the residency disturbing. I was so antsy I even helped deliver grocery coupons a few times. Nancy had gotten the job when we first came back to Columbus to help make money and when she wasn't able to deliver, I filled in. I remember the look of horror on the face of Steve Peters's wife when I handed her their bag of coupons on the front porch. I don't know why she was so shocked. It was still a delivery.

Solo practice was an ideal setup for overworking myself. For better or worse, I could do what I wanted with the schedule. When I took over Schmidt's practice, I left OSU's University Hospital and began working at St. Ann's because it was the local community hospital in the Westerville suburb and it was where Schmidt had practiced. Then I added Grant for the excitement, the teaching, and, yes, the money. So for the years I spent trying to buy out Schmidt, I worked days at my office, saw patients at St. Ann's, worked nights at Grant and did one day a week in the Grant clinic. Two full-time jobs plus the clinic work. That continued when I went to George's and then I added two half-days each week at the St. Ann clinic. I began to phase out Grant, but really I just replaced the hours at St. Ann's. It was too much. That was the period in which I had to wear the Holter monitor because my heart rhythms were getting creative. Heart issues are never a good sign when you're overworking. After two years at George's I got a chance to join a group practice. I knew it was the right thing to do.

Steve Devoe was a longtime attending at Riverside Hospital, another suburban community hospital, but one that was just five minutes from our house. Steve and his brother Keith began practicing at Riverside twenty years before and it was a textbook example of a successful practice: big, well-staffed, and beautifully run. At one time they had as many as seven doctors and plenty of nurses and office staff. They were down to three docs at that point, but that meant that I would be on call only every third night instead of every night — a major difference in the use of my time.

Steve scheduled efficiently and billed efficiently. The insurance staff were experts, and the office was in a building next to the hospital. They were smart people and for the first time I could see how a big, community hospital practice should be run. That was clear when I got there and asked for an ultrasound machine. The Devoes were older doctors who had been trained before ultrasound, but a machine was essential to me. Not surprisingly, the prices had only gone up every year. Steve and Keith, though, had joined a large group of practices that gave them a lot of buying power. The ultrasound that cost twenty thousand dollars when I was buying Schmidt's practice was forty thousand by the time I started with Steve. Through the buying group it cost five thousand. For someone — me — who had discovered his lack of business skills the hard way — bankruptcy — working with Steve was eye opening and reassuring. (Did I mention that after my first year of solo practice I found that my accountant hadn't withheld my federal taxes? That was an expensive April.) It was hard to leave George because I liked him and was deeply grateful for the way he had rescued me. But two practices and two contrasting styles in that small space were a tight fit. More importantly, I needed to think about Nancy and the kids and my relationship to my family.

So I dropped Grant and started seeing Riverside patients along with my St. Ann's patients. And because of Riverside's location near our house, I could spend more time at home. There were times when I got a call from Riverside, met my patient at the hospital, delivered her baby, and was home again in less than an hour. I spent five years working with Steve and it was a good time for Nancy and me. I was at home more and when I was at work I was enjoying it more. It's amazing how your perspective changes when you're rested. Riverside and St. Ann's were similar community hospitals and I love that environment. In addition to all that, I was able to teach residents at St. Ann's. The years working with Steve Devoe were among the best I've had. There had been other highs, but they were different. I experienced sheer joy when I first practiced solo, a feeling unlike anywhere else, a sense of freedom and possibility that working with someone else, or certainly *for* someone else, can't match. But I abused that freedom. With Steve I was able to do good work with families I knew, assist less fortunate patients in the St. Ann's clinic, and continue to teach. Most importantly, I could reclaim my family life.

Maybe it was because I finally had time to think or maybe it was because I saw what a sensible schedule was doing for the Kington family, but whatever the reason, an idea started to form about a way to avoid overworking and do more of what had become my first love, teaching. I was going back and forth from Riverside to St. Ann's and doing both private and clinical practice. What if I gave up my private practice and became an in-house attending for the hospital? That would put an attending physician right there on the floor for any hospital patient whether she was a clinic patient with no outside doctor or a private patient whose attending wasn't immediately available. The hours would be regular, and I could do all the teaching of the residents. Today that sort of doctor is common in hospitals and is called a laborist; then it was something new.

So I went to Karen Robeano, St. Ann's vice president of Nursing, and told her that she needed another employee. Karen liked the idea and took it to the administration. The lawyers made it clear that it would be illegal to keep any private patients so as to eliminate even the perception of favoritism to a staff doctor. I understood that. It was difficult to say goodbye to my longtime patients and to Steve Devoe, too. I placed the patients with some great colleagues, and Steve took it in stride. Moving is part of modern medicine. After twenty years of practice, I became the first laborist at St. Ann's.

It was the best professional decision I ever made. I was teaching a lot and working with a mix of patients admitted from the clinic and under the care of other attendings. But I was the guy who, during the day, was always there. It was an ideal situation for me. Like a lot of things in life, of course, ideal situations can change in a hurry. After six months the wheels came off and I was suddenly overworking even more than ever. Here's what happened.

The art of medicine is complicated by the business of it. Perhaps that's always been true to some extent, but it's especially so these days. The independent hospital is nearly extinct. Hospitals now are part of large corporate systems that determine policies and practices. St. Ann's doctors had been teaching Riverside ob-gyn residents for years even though the hospitals were in different systems — in business terms, they were competitors. It was an unusual arrangement. There were only three Riverside OB residents, but it worked well. The St. Ann's program was small, but good. Then it was gone. The corporation that owned Riverside decided that the arrangement wasn't good business and pulled their residents. That meant that we at St. Ann's weren't just short-staffed, we were unstaffed. Only attending physicians were left to treat patients, and they also had their private practices to run.

As a community hospital, St. Ann's had twenty OBs on staff, but the staffing configuration counts on having residents to help perform over three hundred deliveries a month. It's the residents who take care of things in the middle of the night. They are there for emergencies. It becomes difficult for a private attending to manage patients in labor in a hospital with no residents. I was the only doctor staffing the clinic, and I couldn't manage it because I couldn't leave labor and delivery.

So we hired midwives for the clinic and found an attending in Akron — a hundred miles away — who could work two twenty-four hour shifts on Wednesdays and Sundays. Phil Garner was even older than I was and was an interesting guy. He had gone to med school in Mexico and the Mexican national soccer team practiced right across the road from the hospital. Phil was a very good soccer player, and at some point he crossed the road and talked to the coaches about playing. They gave him a tryout and, as a resident of the country, he ended up on the Mexican Olympic soccer team. I can't imagine doing that during med school. Phil is a bright guy, and we were lucky to get him.

In addition to Phil, we got the rest of the attendings to pitch in. Talk about workaholism. We had doctors in their offices all day Thursday who came in after their office hours and worked all Thursday night, who then went back and did their regular office hours on Friday. They did thirty-six hour shifts and some did two night shifts a week. I was filling a lot of holes and too easily slipped back into full workaholic mode. Well, I'd laid down heavy ruts in that track by overworking for decades and hadn't gotten the vehicle free of them for too long. The wheels slid right back into those ruts with barely a lurch.

We approached Ohio State about sending us residents. They were reluctant, but thank God we had a good negotiator. Phil Shubert was a Maternal Fetal Medicine attending who was recently on the OSU staff, still knew a lot of people over there, and was running interference for us. It was a tricky situation. St. Ann's was part of the Mount Carmel hospital system and Mount Carmel West Hospital was already using Ohio State OB residents even though the hospitals were in competing systems. Now that we at St. Ann's wanted OSU residents, the politics were becoming crazy complicated. Ohio State was already providing a competitor with residents. Was it wise for them to provide even more to another hospital? And was Mount Carmel risking its quota of residents? On the other hand, Mount Carmel was doing ninety deliveries a month and had nine residents. St. Ann's was doing three hundred a month and had no residents. How could those patients get adequate care?

Having no residents, of course, meant that we had no director of residents to handle the negotiations. Phil wanted to be director once we got some residents. St. Ann's really was the red-headed stepchild among the three hospitals, and Phil had a hell of a time working through all the problems and politics, but he got it done. In 2006, two years after the ordeal began, OSU finally agreed to send one resident. The next year they sent us two, and the year after that, three. By 2010, we had a full staff of six residents — an intern and a second-year during the day, two third-years, a chief, and a night float. The nightmare was over.

As the residents drifted in one by one, I was so grateful that I felt a real tendency to coddle them. It would have been so natural to ease up on these life-saving residents — life saving to me, I mean — to relieve them of some of the hardship and stress all residents must work through, and to give them no reason to leave. Ever. Maybe I could buy a giant padlock for the hospital gates? But my job as the director of teaching was to challenge them in ways that forced them to make their own connections and to have their own insights. To do that, the effective teacher uses the Socratic Method — asking questions and trying not to answer them.

During one C-section, Jeanne, one of those new OSU residents, and I opened the patient and saw a huge mass. It was the size of a volleyball. We couldn't see the uterus and so, of course, we couldn't see the baby. Jeanne was confused and didn't know what to do. I had an idea of what the problem was and a glance at the floor confirmed it, but I kept pulling her toward the answer.

"The mass looks like it's filled with fluid," I said, "So we could put a needle in and drain it so you could see. But we have to make sure it's not an ovary and not malignant. What other organs are in this location that it might be?"

Jeanne said, "The only thing I can think of is the bladder. But her bladder's empty. She's got a Foley in it." Jeanne was talking about a Foley catheter.

"Yeah, that's what I was thinking. It sure looks like a bladder and it's in the right place for a bladder. Is the Foley the only reason it couldn't be?"

"Yes, I guess so."

"What if the Foley's not working?"

She thought about that for a moment then followed the Foley tube all the way to the floor, where her foot stood on it. In the short time since we started the section, the blocked drainage tube had backed up enough urine to distend the bladder. We had a good laugh about it. Jeanne was embarrassed, but there was no reason to be. She'd never seen a bladder that wasn't drained before, but I had and I knew this one wasn't draining. That kind of thing is so simple — after you go through years of getting it wrong. Even after I had been practicing for twenty years there were still things I saw and had no idea what I was looking at. It's amazing how different pathologic conditions and anatomies can appear.

Perhaps teaching a resident by not supplying the answers might seem mean-spirited, but it's really the most effective way to do it. Besides, if I had really wanted to be mean I could have let her put the needle into the bladder. It wouldn't have hurt the bladder, and she would have received a lifelong lesson about sticking needles into things you don't recognize.

Another problem C-section and another Foley story. A resident had opened a patient and was looking at mucosa — mucus membrane — that she couldn't recognize. She said, "Are we in the bladder? This looks like bladder."

"It does. It's mucosa, like the bladder. But doesn't the bladder have a Foley bulb in it? Can you find the Foley bulb?"

She felt around for the Foley bulb and couldn't find it. So she went looking. The area was wide open, and she reached her hand in until it disappeared along with most of her forearm. Way down into whatever it was she felt the tube of the Foley.

"That can't be the bladder," I told her, "because the Foley can't be that far away."

In turned out that her arm was in the vagina and the mucosal surface was the vaginal wall. Her hand had gone through the vagina and was between the patient's legs. That's where she felt the Foley tube. The bulb was back where it should have been in the bladder. Maybe this kind of disorientation sounds unbelievable or incompetent to an outsider, but it's neither. It's that same old matter of learning to see what's in front of you. And opening your eyes doesn't do much unless you mentally open up the possibilities the situations present. Don't decide what you *couldn't* be looking at before you interrogate yourself completely.

Besides the physical anatomy of a patient, which can be hard enough to recognize and navigate, there's a mental anatomy. This anatomy resides in the doctor's head and is a mixture of textbook illustrations, med school models, cadaver work, electronic scans, and experience. If the doctor remains in that mental anatomy, it's easy to get lost. We have to break out of it through experience — experience enough to ignore everything but what's right there, and sometimes part of what you must ignore is previous experience. Maybe that idea sounds like Zen mysticism, but it has consequences that are practical at a life-or-death level. That's the thing I love most about teaching--being there when the seeing starts. Don't think, though, that it's only residents who get disoriented inside a patient's body. It can happen to anyone and to whole groups of anyones. Those are the stories we call "Where's the Baby?"

Chapter 13

Where's the Baby?

In Which Infants Throw Surprise Parties

Sometimes I think I've spent most of my career trying to figure out where the baby is — usually in the first trimester when you're wondering if it's in the tubes or in the uterus. But there have been a few times when a full-term baby got lost. Does that sound surprising or even careless? It happens to the best of doctors.

I got an early education in disappearing babies while I was still a resident at St. Francis. We had a patient who was religious about coming to the clinic. When she was thirty-seven weeks she asked if she could travel to South Carolina to visit family. We said no. She was too far along — just three weeks from her due date. Too many things can happen at that late date, and too many of them aren't good. Then she disappeared. That happens all the time. We just shrugged and figured she went to South Carolina. After she missed her next two appointments we wrote her off.

Ten weeks later she arrived in the ER with quite a story. Yes, she had gone south to see her family and decided that she was going to deliver down there. Her due date came and went, though, and after two weeks she had terrible pain and went into the hospital. The doctors examined her, told her that everything was okay, but that she should be induced. She didn't want that, so she went home and, eventually, the pain went away.

Six weeks after her due date she got back to Hartford, and a week after that she came into our ER. She was at forty-seven weeks now and thought that she should have her baby, but she just wasn't going into labor. The ER sent her to us, and we scanned her. I found a thigh bone in the scan and could hear a heartbeat so, as hard as it was to believe, she was still pregnant. There was no more time for her to choose, however, so we started Pitocin to induce her. Nothing happened. Nothing happened all night. I finally went home about midnight. When I came back in the next morning she was still being induced and hadn't dilated one centimeter.

This case began shaping what I call The Kington Principles. Kington Principle 1: If you have trouble inducing labor, consider the possibility that the baby is not in the uterus. At that point, though, the light bulb had not gone on. We knew that we were dealing with a weird uterus, because she'd been carrying for forty-seven weeks. That probably explained it. Now it was clear that we had to perform a C-section.

When we entered the abdomen we saw what looked like two-thirds of a uterus on the right, the other third on the left, and an umbilical cord — still merrily pulsing — snaking off into the abdomen and disappearing into the bowels. There's that question. Where's the baby? It's at the end of that umbilical cord, of course, but the intestines were stuck to it in lots of nasty adhesions — scar tissue only partially healed. This mess was something that hadn't happened recently. There had been some sort of catastrophe weeks earlier.

We carefully dissected our way along the adhered intestines until we got them off the umbilical cord and finally found the baby up under the liver. It was like a little old man, wrinkled and emaciated, but still alive. After piecing together the patient's story, we decided that the terrible pain she felt in South Carolina was the uterus splitting in two. Then she stopped bleeding. In my limited experience, I had never heard of that happening after such trauma and that's still the only time I've run across it in the many years since. The little guy did beautifully, though. He was in the NICU for a few weeks but responded well to nursing care. Once we were able to feed him with something better than an overstressed umbilical cord, he thrived. It was remarkable that he lived seven weeks beyond due date. Even forty-three to forty-four week babies generally don't make it. It's even more remarkable that he exited the uterus and lived. Usually those mothers bleed so much that they are likely to die, and their baby almost certainly does.

It may seem incredible that a baby could end up under the liver, but once a baby leaves the uterus the abdomen provides some frustrating hiding places. I worked with an attending who will remain nameless, because he had earned a bad reputation for working too quickly. There's quick and efficient and there's quick and out on the golf course, and this guy was in the second group. Sometimes he started stitching the uterus closed before the placenta had delivered so he didn't have to waste any time waiting. One night he was delivering a baby and as he was lifting out the head it slid up and over the top of the uterus and into the abdomen. Instead of delivering the baby south, he delivered it north into the mother's body. The uterus was so big that he couldn't simply pull the baby out. He had to deliver the placenta, shrink the uterus, then go in and get the baby. I thought that the doctor's habit of rushing probably caused the problem. I don't know if he's slowed down, but I haven't heard of him losing another baby.

A sad case of a disappearing baby happened at St. Ann's. Scans had told us that the mother had twins, but once we had removed a large cyst there was only one baby in the uterus. We were trying to figure out where the other twin had gone when the tray where we had placed the cyst began to shake. We took a closer look and it was the other baby — an acardiac twin, small, born without a heart, and with an amniotic sac so thick and deformed that we hadn't recognized it as one. Reflexes caused the movement that alerted us. It was unnerving and like any birth anomaly, depressing. Acardiac twins are rare, I'm glad to say — about one in thirty-five thousand births.

I remember another "Where's the Baby?" at St. Ann's with a happy outcome. I had a soft spot for Ron Roberts, a second-year resident, because he had five kids, too. Ron had come in for morning rounds and was standing at the nurse's station looking at the room readouts.

"Where's the baby in room four? It's not on the monitor anymore."

Everyone stared up at the monitor and he was right. What had been a set of healthy readings just minutes earlier was gone. Ron rushed into room four and the mother was asleep. He brushed away the tubes, lowered the side rail and threw back the sheet. There, sleeping peacefully between the mother's legs, was her newborn son. She'd had what we call a "dense" epidural for pain, a substantial dose, and was knocked out. She told Ron that she remembered coughing once and figured that was when she delivered.

In the early days of ultrasound, it was easier to lose a baby because it was harder to read a scan. At St. Francis when Craig Huttler was a resident and Rick Fortuna was chief, they scanned a big woman who looked like she could be carrying twins. The chief had been called in because of the twins. The scan was murky, but they were sure they saw two babies. So they placed two fetal heart monitors on the patient's belly and, sure enough, there were the two little hearts beating away. They delivered the first baby, clamped the cord, then went to break the bag of waters on the second baby. But there was no bag. There was no second baby. They thought that there were twins so that's what they saw on the blurry ultrasounds. When they looked at the heart monitor tracings they realized that they were notably similar, because they were reading the same heart. That case is another example of needing to see what you're looking at.

Craig had a different case with a tragic outcome. A young woman drove into the St. Francis lot at high speed, her family right behind her in another car, and she slammed into the ER canopy. Craig was just leaving the ER after checking a possible ectopic when he heard a commotion in the trauma room. The whole family was in there and the mother was screaming, "Save the baby! Save the baby!" Her daughter had severe head damage and wasn't going to survive. The trauma team was keeping her alive because the family was telling them that she was full-term and the baby had to be saved. So when they saw Craig walking by they grabbed him and told him he needed to do a stat C-section on the patient.

She was a big woman, too, and Craig was dealing with those primitive ultrasounds. He couldn't see much, so he asked for a scalpel and did a C-section. It didn't take long. A post-mortem section is easy to do, because there's no bleeding. But when Craig looked inside he saw a normal-sized uterus. The young woman wasn't pregnant. Never had been. The family was stunned, of course, and refused to believe it at first. After nine months of happy expectations who would be willing to believe it was all a lie? The situation isn't unheard of. Women may fake a pregnancy in an attempt to get attention, as a way to manipulate a partner, or in an effort to feel better about oneself or delude oneself. The tragic outcome of this case was unforgettable, though.

I've wondered many times since then what might have happened if the family hadn't followed behind so closely. Maybe if the patient could have entered the hospital by herself, she might have had a chance to convince them of a miscarriage. In full emotional crisis, though, with a carful of people trailing right behind her, driving into the building might have seemed her only choice. Did she expect to survive? Could she blame a miscarriage on the accident? Would the disorder of an accident mask the false story? Those are questions I will never get out of my head.

I hope that telling "Where's the Baby?" stories doesn't diminish the competence of ob-gyns in your eyes. To me, the stories are not about the competence of the doctors as much as the endless surprises provided by the human body. As I learned during my first term in med school, the same organs can look confusingly different in different patients. Even their locations can vary between patients, and, yes, the medical technology we use to follow a pregnancy has become far better. Today, ultrasound technology is so good that doctors know immediately if the patient has an acardiac twin. There are other variables, though. It matters how many babies you're looking at and how far along in the pregnancy they are. Doctors have ended up not with fewer babies than they expected, but with more.

We had a case of quadruplets at St. Ann's in the early nineties, and those were the days when that was not as common as fertility medicine has made it. They were natural quadruplets, and they'd been followed carefully for months. When it was time for them to deliver, the newspaper and TV reporters came, and there was a huge amount of publicity. The hospital had four incubators with two NICU nurses at each one and all the assembled OBs were there ready for assistance and photo ops. It was a big production. I was standing in the doorway watching everything, because it was too crowded in the delivery room for me to squeeze in.

The babies hadn't been named yet, so they were calling them "A" and "B" as they came out and were placed into incubator "A," "B," and so forth. Then I saw Larry Polito, the attending in charge, with his hand still in the mom's abdomen. Larry paused, and I saw his eyes above the mask widen.

"There's another one."

Out came baby E. They didn't have an extra incubator so little E had to double up with a sibling. All those months they had been scanning the babies and thought there were four, but it's hard to keep them separated sometimes. Today such a thing is less likely because ultrasounds for multiple births are done much earlier. That mother probably had her first scan at fourteen to fifteen weeks. Now it's at six.

These days, when you've got what's called "assisted reproductive technology" and you've got five or eight babies in there you see them when they're tiny. You can get all, or most of them, on the screen at the same time. Once they're bigger and you can only get part of a baby on the screen, it's harder to know whether you're scanning the same one. By the third trimester you're only looking at parts. When you're studying one heart and you go to look at another one, you'd better go directly there if you can. If you wander, it's possible to circle back to the same heart.

Modern digital ultrasound machines allow the doctor to freeze the screen, then drag a cursor across it to measure an organ or a bone. Sometimes you'll measure a thighbone and you'll think "That's the same length that I measured before." You've probably got the same baby, so you need to keep comparing to make sure. Dragging that cursor is easy, but it's harder to know if you've got the left thighbone of baby A or the right thighbone of baby B.

I was measuring the parts of a baby one time and pointing out his anatomy to the very young mother beside me.

"Here's an arm," I said, "and here's a leg." "Here's the head."

She turned to me and said,

"When do they all get put together?"

I didn't have an answer for that one. It's evidence, though, of how our mysterious and miraculous bodies can look so confusing as we delve inside them. That can be true of a seventeen-year-old mother or a trained physician who ends up asking,

"Where's the baby?"

Chapter 14

Nurses

In Which I Realize the Importance of RNs

I love nurses. It's no secret — Nancy knows. You have to love someone who chooses a career taking care of others — a career where the pay isn't great, the hours are long, and the work is stressful and physically difficult. Early in my residency when I began seeing what labor and delivery nurses had to do, I was very glad I was a doctor and not one of them. The L and D nurse has to assist the patient from early labor to delivery, keep both the mother and baby safe, keep the family at bay, and clean up all the mess. And with a birth there is a lot of mess. The blood that's such a part of our world is cleaned up by the nurse. The doctor just has to order an enema. It's the nurse who has to give it. Labor is a difficult and emotionally charged process. In birth we generally see women at their best, but sometimes at their worst. The nurse has to deal with all of that. The doctor is often sitting at home waiting for the phone call telling him to come in and catch the baby.

There's an old hospital joke about an unidentified body that's found in a river. The police are trying to identify it and they figure it must be a nurse because the bladder is full, the stomach is empty, and there are scars all over the butt from being chewed out. Nurses have bailed me out many times and I really appreciate it. There are bad ones, just like there are bad doctors, but they're rare, and if a doctor has a good nurse it makes all the difference in the world. I've seen nurses save patients, and their doctors, from disaster.

I remember one family practice resident who was doing his first delivery and was nervous and tentative. Nervous is okay. Tentative is not. A doctor has to be able to make a decision in a moment, and a mother or baby's life may depend on it being the right one. We had a salty old-timer as our head nurse, and she looked at me and rolled her eyes at the way that green resident was working. Finally, he delivered the baby, put it up on the mother's abdomen, clamped the umbilical cord, then took the scissors and cut below the clamp. There was a little nub of an umbilical cord left, about a quarter of an inch. I snatched it before it retracted and disappeared.

"You cut below the clamp! Put another clamp on that!"

He had an astonished, confused look on his face and instead of reaching for another clamp he brought the scissors up and moved in to cut the cord again. I didn't even have time to yell, but in a split second the nurse made a half-turn, cocked her right arm, and smashed that resident right in the sternum. He staggered backwards from the force of the thump and gust from her roar.

"Get out of the way!"

Then she reached over to the tray, got the clamp herself, and made sure the umbilical cord was tied.

When I was in my residency, nurses helped me out constantly, and I learned early to ask for their opinions. Checking the dilation of a patient in labor is a skill that has to be learned over time. You use your fingers to see how much the cervix is dilated, but at first it's hard to gauge what you're feeling. Young doctors have to do it dozens of times before they know what they're doing. I got used to querying the nurse and getting corrected.

"Is she three centimeters?"

"More like eight."

The residents who come in with a chip on their shoulder and treat the nurse like an underling are missing a great resource and damaging their own learning process. They're also not very popular with the experienced nurses who know a lot more than they do. Actually, doctors can behave like jerks.

One cocky resident I knew was awakened in the call room by a nurse.

"I think this patient is pretty active. I need you to get in here and check her."

The resident let out a big sigh and came down the hall with his chest out and all his body language communicating his displeasure with being disturbed. He checked the patient, turned with disgust to the nurse and said, "She's only two centimeters! Don't call me again until she's actually ready to deliver."

He got about halfway to the door when a baby's butt started to crown out of the mother. The patient had been ten centimeters, but it was a breech birth and the resident had been feeling the baby's rear instead of the mother's cervix.

The nurse wasn't going to let him escape that one and said, "Congratulations, Doctor. You've just given this boy his first rectal exam."

That sort of thing can be hard to live down.

The good nurses are good at a lot of things, including hospital politics. They can guide the green residents and also know when to go to the attendings and tell them that the resident is making a mistake. That's so valuable because no one sees as much of a patient as the nurse does. No one knows the patient better. It's a point I stress now when I teach Crew Resource Management. The most important history is the history of the person who's with the patient the most. They know what's going on. The doctor doesn't have the whole picture like the nurse who's been there for hours. One of the most important things I can do as a teacher is to get the resident to listen to the nurse. Listening to the patient is crucial; listening to the nurse is just as crucial.

The workload of nurses has only gotten worse in the past decade because now they have to comply with electronic medical records laws that demand hours of computer time logging case information. Because of all the things they are called upon to do already, those computer hours are spent after their regular shift is over. When they're dog tired and their scrubs are covered with blood and who knows what, they have to sit at the keyboard and enter the day's records.

The new regulations have changed the role of the nurse as well. There are drug protocols now that specify the medications and dosages to be used in particular situations. Because of that, a nurse might be administering Pitocin to a patient under the guidance of a regulation instead of the guidance of a doctor. That puts the nurse in the middle of very important decisions that she or he might be uncomfortable about.

Any hospital, no matter how small, is a bureaucracy — with all the burdens and annoyances that bureaucracy brings. It's not always possible, for instance, to get the right number of people on the right unit at the right time. There's always an element of chance involved in figuring out the patient load. I watched a hospital administrator walk onto a unit and demonstrate a lack of knowledge bordering on incompetence.

"Why are all these nurses sitting around doing nothing?"

It happened to be a slow time, so it did look as if we had too much staff. That can change in a second, though, and suddenly you're understaffed. If you ask a charge nurse how many people she or he needs, it's always about twice what the vice president of Nursing thinks is needed. It's a rare moment in which nurses can sit around, and boy, did that comment tick the nurses off.

Rightly so. The administrator was their boss, so they didn't say anything. They sure said something to me.

Labor and delivery nurses love babies, of course, and since the majority of the nurses are women, it's no surprise that there are a lot of nurses having babies themselves. Of course many men who are nurses have the experience of accompanying their partners through childbirth, but right now I'm talking about the women and they tend to be a pretty hardy bunch. They've seen a lot of births and the pain, the blood, and the uncertainty are familiar to them.

There was a night during my residency when three nurses were on the floor in the last stage of their pregnancies, all pushing at the same time. Kenny Fratiane was their attending and he knew he wasn't going to be able to be at each delivery, so he brought me in. That was a good idea because they all delivered within two minutes of each other. I delivered two, and Kenny delivered one. It was a memorable night, but not memorable enough for a guy who's as bad with names as I am. A year later I was introduced to a nurse and told her that I was glad to meet her.

"Well, you've met me before," she said. "You delivered my baby."

I worked with one nurse, Amy, who was very pregnant with her fifth baby. It was the middle of the night, and we were keeping an eye on a problem patient. I went in to check the patient and the nurse wasn't there. I asked where she was, but no one seemed to know. Then she showed up and that peek-a-boo routine kept on for a few hours. It turned out that Amy was in labor herself while working the night shift. She thought her water had broken so she kept going into the bathroom to check. When her shift was over Amy admitted herself, called her doctor, and told him she was five centimeters and ready to deliver. That's toughness. It's good to have that kind of person working beside you in the delivery room when things go south.

I had a patient who was seen in the clinic up until her due date. The last measurement on the resident's chart was forty-four centimeters which is about four centimeters higher than you'd expect it to be at term. She got to the hospital in a rip-roaring labor, pushed for about twenty minutes, and shoved out about half of the biggest head on a baby I've ever seen. Then he got stuck. It's called a shoulder dystocia — the baby's shoulders get caught on the mother's pelvic bones. Informally, it's called a "turtle sign" because the head sticks out then tucks back in like a turtle.

This condition dictates about five or six specific maneuvers to try, but basically what you've got is a lot of twisting and turning going on with the doctor being careful not to pull too hard because the nerves in the baby's shoulders can be damaged. The resident went through the maneuvers in order and finally got to the Zavenelli maneuver, which most doctors only see on reruns of ER. That's a last-ditch effort where you try to put the baby's head back in. That didn't work, so I switched places with him and I couldn't budge the kid either. I told Amy that we needed to get the mother to the OR, and she did the magic trick that I've seen good nurses do hundreds of times — got the patient placed comfortably, totally unplugged, bedrails safely up, rolled out and moving down the hall in a matter of seconds. Take my word for it; that's hard to do. She was probably thinking the same thing I was, which was "what the hell are we going to do when we get her there?"

That was the point at which Fast Eddie stepped in. We had a medical student who, until then, was simply called Eddie, but he decided to help out on this tough delivery and beat us all to the OR and took my gown and gloves. I admired his initiative, but I didn't have time to get out a new set of gloves and gown, so I just poured betadine on the patient's abdomen, grabbed a scalpel barehanded, and did a laparotomy.

I didn't take the time to make an incision in the uterus; when I got inside I pushed down on the baby's anterior shoulder while the resident pulled from below.

"I think it's coming! I think it's coming! No. No … it's not coming."

So we switched places, and he pushed from above while I pulled from below. That went on for two minutes that seemed like two hours. The situation was frustrating, and the longer it went on the more dangerous it was becoming. We had to get that baby unstuck or it was going to die. Without any alternative, I grabbed the little guy's shoulder, broke it in my hand, and twisted him out.

We sent him up to Neonatal Intensive Care. And he, at twelve pounds two ounces, sat in an incubator with a cast on his arm next to the three-pound preemies. It was quite a sight. His shoulder healed quickly and when he came back for a checkup at six weeks, everything was fine. He looked like he should be entering first grade.

That birth was a nightmare, but Amy made it far easier than it might have been. That's what a good nurse does. She went through every step with us — applied suprapubic pressure; climbed up on the patient trying to push the shoulder through; pulled back the baby's legs; pushed the mother's legs up against her body in a McRoberts maneuver. And getting us down to the OR so quickly and efficiently was all Amy. By the time we rolled in there, she had already lined up the patient care techs and circulating nurses for a C-section, called anesthesia, transferred the patient to a delivery bed, and managed to get her mask and bonnet on. It was seven and a-half minutes from the moment the baby got stuck until we delivered him. That's really fast. Because it happened on March 17th I still call this case the St. Patrick's Day Massacre, but really it was a complete success and that couldn't have happened without a great nurse. By the way, Eddie was Fast Eddie for the rest of med school.

A year later the patient came back in for a checkup and a different nurse did her intake interview.

"Was your son's birth a vaginal delivery or a C-section?"

"Both."

The nurse managed not to laugh and went to find Amy.

"Well, she sort of *did* have both ..."

There are thousands of Amys and their male nurse counterparts working in hospitals all over the country. If you ask me all of them, in every specialty, deserve medals — though they'd probably rather have a raise. Anyone who wants to say something bad about nurses had better not say it to me, and Nancy is in wholehearted agreement with that.

Chapter 15

Good, Bad, and Ugly

In Which I Face Changes of All Sorts

I suppose that if you looked at any thirty-year stretch of medical history you would see some remarkable changes. In the thirty years since I entered it, though, the practice of medicine has been absolutely transformed.

Some of the biggest changes, of course, are technological, and perhaps the biggest of those has been the move from handwritten notes and charts to the electronic medical record. The electronic record sounds like a wonderful idea. It's legible, so it should minimize mistakes; it's thorough, since it prompts its writers if they forget anything; it's sharable, so if someone has a medical emergency on vacation in Florida they can get their record sent from Cleveland. The concept sounds wonderful. But it just doesn't work that way. I think it's turned out to be a horrible development because it places a computer between the patient and the doctor or nurse.

It used to be that when you went in to see a patient in labor, the nurse was at the bedside monitoring the baby or the patient's contractions — maybe helping her walk around, or bounce on a ball, or get in a tub. Any number of useful, hands-on things were happening. Now when you walk into a room invariably the nurse has her back to the patient and is furiously typing away at the keyboard trying to get everything documented. When doctors do a delivery these days, they spend about ten or fifteen minutes with the mother and baby and a half hour with the computer. I'd say that the people deserve more attention than the machine does.

The influence of that machine goes deeper than that. Many times I've seen doctors sit down at a computer and try to do something and the computer won't let them do it. They might be trying to prescribe a medicine, but if it's not the medicine that the computer *thinks* is being prescribed, the doctor can't enter it correctly. So doctors will change their orders based on what the machine will allow them to enter and the patient ends up with their doctor's second-best choice.

The computerized chart is probably four or five times as long as the handwritten chart was. It has reams of useless information, and doctors or nurses have to wade through all of it if they want to do a careful job. Every patient has her sheet of social work or discharge planning or who knows what. Most of our patients are healthy young women who are having a baby and are going home, so the discharge plan could be simply "go home and enjoy your baby." You can push thoroughness until it becomes inefficiency.

There also have been some major advances in surgery that I've mentioned along the course of my story. When I was a resident, if you had an ectopic pregnancy you had a laparotomy, were in the hospital three days, and recovered for six weeks. Now you can have a laparoscopy, go home the same day, and recover for a week. Or you can take a medicine and not have surgery at all.

Robotic surgery is also a powerful change. With laparoscopy the doctor's hands are working the controls of a robot and the robotic hands instead of the doctor's hands are inside the abdomen working the inserted cutting and tying instruments. Sound complicated? Yeah. It's also expensive.

The upside is that the little robotic fingers can be faster and get into narrower places. That's why, in some cases, it's a great tool to have. There are times that the doctor needs to get somewhere in the patient's abdomen that he or she couldn't otherwise get to. That's a small number of cases, though.

Now medical groups are putting up billboards advertising their robotic surgery and building a demand among patients. That's another major change in medicine since I began. Then you couldn't advertise anything. Now ads are all over the place, and I think it's another negative development. Patients are entitled to have thoughtful care that's tailored to them; they shouldn't be shoehorned into a procedure because that's what the doctor likes to do. Somebody once said that invention is the mother of necessity, and in medicine that's not necessarily good for the patient.

And these days the pharmaceutical companies are constantly barraging people with the idea that they need a medicine and they should talk to their doctor about it. That's the wrong way around. Doctors should tell patients what they need, not the opposite. An informed patient with an opinion is a good thing — even a valuable thing. Do you think the patient is being fairly informed by drug ads? Not me.

Sometimes I hear doctors criticized for being manipulated by drug companies through fancy meals or junkets. Those days are long gone. That sort of thing became heavily restricted by the federal government, and good for them. Then advertising restrictions were lifted and now the pharmaceutical people don't need to send docs to a Red Sox game; they aim their money at the consumer. Before, doctors could watch the game and still prescribe what they wanted. The patient is actually harder to resist because the doctor can lose them.

There's also the questionable practice of doctors being paid for research on medical equipment. Some orthopedic surgeons just got a lot of publicity for receiving over a million dollars a year from a company that makes artificial joints. Research is a fine thing, but it's got to be awfully rough to use a competitor's better hip when you're getting two million dollars a year from someone else.

The supervision of residency programs has changed completely and that's created what I'm doing now at the end of my career. When I started out, residents all had an attending physician, but he or she wasn't in the hospital and if you were operating, as in my first vaginal hysterectomy, the attending might be outside in the lounge reading a paper. You can't do that now. The attending has to be in the operating room from fascia to fascia — from opening the abdomen to closing it. For vaginal deliveries they have to be there for the majority of the procedure. Put simply, attendings now actually have to be in attendance. Back in the old days the resident usually called in the attending from home and that was usually after they had gotten themselves into some trouble. I think having the attending in attendance is a big improvement in safety and education.

In private practice I was teaching as much as I could, but attendings were able to cover from their offices or homes and everybody was signing up to cover the residents but not really being there. That was how the residents were educated — from the doc they could call. Now, since those attendings can't take time away from their office, the responsibility of teaching falls to doctors like me who are already there in the hospital for the very purpose of teaching and supervising residents. So as my solo practice started to wind down, I took a job from the hospital because they needed an attending who was present all the time to teach.

There is one change, though, that has been the most corrosive and damaging to the practice of medicine over the last thirty years and that is the impact of medical litigation. Malpractice lawsuits have fundamentally altered the way doctors and hospitals do their work, and not for the better. Useful drugs and procedures have been abandoned and often we are forced to tiptoe through a patient's therapy. That's not good for patient or doctor.

I know that there are bad doctors. I've seen some over the years, and I want them to pay for their mistakes. I want them gone. I also know that some drugs can be dangerous if they're not used carefully and intelligently. I'm not against lawyers. Hospitals employ swarms of them, and we couldn't get along without them. My brother is a lawyer, and I mentioned how he helped me. I've seen what's happened to medicine because of unbridled litigation, though, and it's disturbing.

Doctors have been talking since I was in my residency about how the ambulance chasers have ruined things, so the problem has been growing for a long time. The old-timers used to talk about how it's perfectly safe to do a breech delivery, but no one does them anymore. The same is true of forceps delivery. Those are dying arts in obstetrics, and the skill of the doctor is the key to both. It's definitely riskier when a baby is delivered butt first. What most people don't know is that the only option, the C-section, is as risky as the breech birth. There is twice the risk of the mother dying. There are about three maternal deaths per ten thousand vaginal deliveries and around six for C-sections. But nobody gets sued for doing a C-section.

C-sections have become so commonplace that the risk is overlooked. In Brazil they're doing elective C-sections now. We've avoided that, but our C-section rate is about thirty-five percent. The best studies I saw when I was a resident said that the true rate of unavoidable C-section births should be about five to seven percent. The rate has drifted up and up over the years, and I think it's mainly because of legal considerations.

In addition to these useful procedures we've lost some effective drugs. Bendectin was wonderful for combating the nausea and vomiting of morning sickness. A combination of vitamin B6 and an antihistamine, it had been around since the mid-50s, and there were never any epidemiological studies that found that it caused birth defects. Yet its manufacturer stopped selling it in 1983 because of lawsuits that asserted that it did. One of the most famous Bendectin lawsuits was led by the celebrity attorney Melvin Belli. His primary witness was later found to have falsified the research he cited, and even though the FDA never found any evidence that the link with birth defects was true, the damage was done. Nancy had regretted the loss of Bendectin even before I got into medicine. She used it for her first two pregnancies and it really helped. By the time our third came along it was gone even though it was perfectly safe.

Pitocin, a hormone used to induce labor and to stop bleeding, is another drug that's been hit with lawsuits. My sister warned me about Pitocin when I was a resident. She was living on the West Coast and sent me an article about the top ten grossing malpractice suits in California. Nine of them involved Pitocin, and she wondered if I knew about this dangerous drug that some OBs were using. I hated to tell her that I used it every day.

Why do we still use it in spite of the lawsuits? Probably because it's indispensable. You can do away with Bendectin and women feel sicker during their pregnancies, but if we did away with Pitocin women would die. That's why the World Health Organization put it on its list of essential drugs. That doesn't stop the lawyers. It's been blamed for uterine ruptures and causing fetal distress by making the labor too strong. It's easy, though, when you're deciding what causes what, to put the cart before the horse. Most of the time when you're using a powerful drug like Pitocin the patient is in a problem pregnancy anyway. If you use Pitocin and get fetal distress, then you should be doing a C-section. If you avoided a C-section and the baby was harmed, it wasn't the Pitocin that harmed the baby. It was probably your delay.

Many crucial medical decisions are made because the doctors are pressed for time and worried about the legal consequences of their decisions. Fatigue and fear are not good reasons for doing important things. If a patient needs to get delivered, for instance, and she's not laboring, then the only choices are to start Pitocin or do a C-section. A lot of doctors are gun shy about Pitocin and just section the patient, and that drives up the maternal mortality rate. It's so much easier for the doctor to do the C-section and that can be seductive. It's the difference between sectioning the patient at 5:00 in the afternoon and running Pitocin until 3:00 in the morning. Especially if you end up having to do a C-section, anyway. That's a tough decision for a doctor who's tired.

If you look at C-section rates, you'll find that a lot of them are done in the early evening and not that many in the wee hours. There's also a bump in the C-section rate after the OB's office is closed. The doctor comes to see the patient to see how she's doing. The doc might have been expecting her to deliver, and now it looks like the delivery might happen at 4:00 in the morning. It's hard to walk away and say, "Call me when you're ready." That's the beauty of the hospital laborist — the OB who's on duty for just such situations. We're there at the hospital and it doesn't matter if we deliver at 4:00 p.m. or at 4:00 a.m. There's no incentive to get the patient delivered before dark.

We can also thank the lawyers for almost bringing back measles. Some people sued because there is a tiny correlation between the measles vaccine and damage to the baby. That ignores the huge correlation between wiping out measles and having healthy babies. The government had to step in and manufacture the vaccine because pharmaceutical companies found it too expensive to defend the lawsuits.

Doctors are practicing defensive medicine now and that's easiest to see in the ER. In the old days when a patient came in with a headache you'd evaluate her, do an H and P, then decide whether to do a CAT scan. Now you get the CAT scan first and evaluate the results. A lot of money is being spent covering doctors' behinds. You don't want to miss anything because you've got that lawyer looking over your shoulder.

We used to be taught that if a patient's headache was her first or her worst to get a CAT scan. Now if someone comes in who's had thirty headaches in her life, and she's got one just like the other twenty-nine she's going to get scanned, even with no neurological symptoms. There's no reason for that.

Litigation has made medical care more expensive, but doctors aren't the ones making those profits. Their income has been shrinking. OBs used to work through March or April to make enough to pay for their malpractice insurance. Now it's more like September or October. Statistically, it's never been safer to have a baby, and it's never been riskier to be a doctor. When something goes wrong *everybody* gets sued. I was involved in a lawsuit that named twelve doctors, the anesthesia department, and the hospital. I was sued once about a patient I had never seen, treated, or written an order for. I was on the chart because I was the one who looked at her pap smear. The pap smear didn't figure in the lawsuit, but my name was there and I got sued.

Litigation drives up costs and insurance companies and hospitals respond by cost cutting. That has resulted in a subtle, but significant change in the philosophy of practice. Hospitals have tried to make medical care uniform, so they now have an approach called "best practice." Doctors across the country are studied to determine the best way to do things. Then those methods are codified and that's the way you are told to do it. Doctors now have very little leeway in treating hospital patients. You have to toe the line, or you'll get a phone call that asks why you didn't use the such-and-such contraption that everyone else is using.

It's a good thing in the sense that it's gotten rid of the outliers who were doing a bad job, but it's also discouraged the outliers who were doing better than everybody else, too. The geniuses and innovators are being forced to do what everybody else does and that's regrettable.

Overall, the practice of medicine in the last thirty years has become far safer for the patient. About ninety-five percent of the time the mother and baby do well. We've made great progress in treating prematurity and delivering babies earlier and earlier. When I was a resident, we'd deliver a twenty-six-week baby and we'd tell the parents that it had about a fifty percent chance to live and about a thirty percent chance to live a normal life. Now we sometimes deliver babies at twenty-three weeks.

The medical profession is facing some significant problems. Something needs to be done about the impact of predatory litigation without weakening the patient's recourse if there's been real harm done. Something needs to be done, as well, to reestablish the human contact that technology is eroding. But I'm proud of my profession as I enter my fourth decade in it. Patients are safer, outcomes are better, and there's still nothing like seeing the joy of a new mother and knowing that we helped make that joy happen.

Chapter 16

Grim Reaper

*In Which I Became the Patient and Get
a Second Medical Education*

I have been frightened in a hospital many times. During my internship that was pretty much the way I lived. As my skills improved, the terror receded, though I was sometimes frightened during the tough cases and at crisis points. That kind of fear, though, was expectable, manageable, and even useful. I never had feared for my own life, and when finally I did, it changed me as a doctor.

In 2008, I decided that it was time to take care of the knee injury I got in 1966. I guess I'm not much of a model for taking care of oneself. After forty-two years I'd had enough. It was bone on bone, and I could no longer golf, ski, or even take a long walk without a lot of pain and swelling the next day. The orthopedic doctor told me I needed a total left knee replacement, so at the beginning of January I made the decision and checked into the hospital. That was the beginning of a harrowing yet invaluable education in what it means to be a patient.

Doctors, in general, don't make very good patients. We diagnose ourselves when we should leave that to others, and we think we have the option of ignoring doctor's orders because we are one. I was probably worse than most. But I had the surgery and it went well. Post-op day one, though, when I was supposed to go home, I began hiccupping — every five seconds all day long. We couldn't get them stopped, and my stay went on from Monday through Saturday. I also had a lot of stomach pain, and if I'd been paying attention I should have been able to diagnose an ulcer. I'm pretty good at ignoring symptoms, though. I made it forty-two years with a shot knee.

After five days and nights I got to the point where I could fall asleep for five-second naps between the hiccups. Finally, they got them stopped, and I went home feeling miserable. But I started to recover and by three weeks out I was doing pretty well. I was off the pain meds and could even drive a car — though I almost had to stand up to do it because I had to keep my left leg straight.

Nancy was terrific as usual and took time off her job until I could manage on my own. After a month, we thought that time had finally come and on her first work morning she headed out and locked the front door behind her. She doesn't remember why, but it was important.

I felt queasy that morning, so I thought I might have a touch of the flu. Even though I wasn't hungry, I decided I should eat so

I had some lunch around 1:00. As soon as I ate I went from queasy to awful and headed for the downstairs bathroom. It's a few steps from the kitchen, which was fortunate, and a few steps from the front door, which turned out to be even better. When I stood I came close to fainting, and I said out loud to no one, "Gosh, I really do have the flu." So I grabbed the crutches and rushed into the bathroom without my cell phone — another small decision with big consequences.

I pulled my crutches into the small bathroom, closed the door, and the next thing I knew was that the left side of my face was really cold. When I opened my eyes I discovered why — it was lying against the bathroom floor. My left leg was up in the air with the foot jammed into the corner and there was a smear of blood running from above the toilet, where I had smashed my face into the wall, all the way down to the cold tiles of the floor. It was covered with all kinds of bodily fluids — just about the whole menu that the human body can manufacture. So being a very logical doctor I said to myself, "Well, it's probably not the flu and I need to get out of here." Then I promptly went to sleep.

When I woke up nothing had changed. No one had rescued me. I was in the same position, and I was starting to realize that I had a big problem. The strangest part was that I really wasn't that interested in solving it. I thought that I might be dying and that was basically okay with me. I could piece together that my death would upset Nancy, though, so I decided to try getting out of there. I took off my t-shirt and mopped some of the mess on the floor so I could have a dry place to push from. Propping myself up, I flipped over and got up onto the toilet. As soon as I did I knew that I was going to faint again, so I dove over to the sink, grabbed a faucet, and tried to stretch out. Now I could stay conscious for a while — about thirty or forty seconds. I decided that I would time how long I was staying awake between faints by counting my pulse. I figured about a hundred and twenty beats per minute would work, but I never got above fifty beats without fainting. It was a silly exercise, but when you're delusional you do silly things and I was getting delusional. Now I understand vividly what blood loss does to the mental process. If I could just hang on, I thought, I could make it. Nancy would probably call me from work to see how I was doing so I just needed to tough out an hour.

I had no idea of the passage of time and even if I could have stayed awake I couldn't have gotten out because my crutches had fallen across the door. Every time I bent over to get them I fainted. I was trapped.

Next I remember hearing the phone ring. I thought vaguely, "Great. Nancy's calling to check on me. Now she'll come home and help me."

Well, it was her, and when I didn't answer she decided that I must have gone out for an ice cream. That was not like her at all. Nancy's kind of a worrier. Luckily for me, she called our daughter Katie in Virginia and told her I wasn't answering the phone and was probably out somewhere.

Katie, who's *not* much of a worrier said, "Mom, what if he's there and he can't answer the phone? Why don't you get a neighbor to check on him?"

So Nancy called Mike next door to come over. I heard the bell and some knocking, and I yelled, "Call 911!"

Since the bathroom was only five or six feet from the front door he heard me. Then I passed out again, and the next thing I remember is the impression that a bunch of people were having some kind of meeting in our kitchen. I began to be concerned that they didn't know where to find me and tried to figure out a way to get their attention. I found out later that they were all crammed into the bathroom doorway and the hall outside talking about what to do with me.

When Nancy pulled into the drive, the EMTs were trying to break into my car so they could open the garage door and make it easier to wheel me out. She opened the door for them and came in just in time to hear one of the guys say, "Well, he's really big and he's really slippery, but I think I can get him."

He could. The guy picked me up and threw me onto the gurney, and I got a glimpse of Nancy behind all the firemen looking worried. To reassure her and thank them I said, "Man, you wouldn't believe how good it feels to be lying down."

He just nodded at me and didn't say anything. That was because, as Nancy told me later, what I really said was along the lines of, "Mangah belayagah fee laladon."

So I was stretched out in the back of the ambulance and Nancy was up in the front seat. The techs were trying to give me an IV, but they couldn't find a vein and I was determined, as a doctor, to guide them through the procedure using my space language. It was all very confused. Nancy thought that because they didn't use their lights or siren I had died back there.

They got the IV in, got me to the hospital, and by the time I rolled through the doors of the ER I was communicating well enough to get into an argument with the ER doc. By the time they got me more or less revived, he came in and said, "Well, Dr. Kington, your hemoglobin is 7.5, but it's our policy not to transfuse anyone until their level is below 7.5. So we're just going to watch you overnight."

That seemed a little rule-happy. It was pretty clear at this point that I had a bleeding ulcer and had lost a lot of blood in the bathroom.

I said, "My hemoglobin three weeks ago was 15. I have high blood pressure and now it's 90 over 40. My pulse is 140. I'm pretty sure my hemoglobin is going to be below 7.5 the next time you check it."

"Yeah, I understand all that," he said, "But we don't know that for a fact. We're going to give you fluids and watch you carefully and see if you need a transfusion."

The guy wouldn't budge, and I started getting a feeling that a lot of patients have — powerlessness. I had a lot of experiences in that hospital stay that made me realize that patients need to have an advocate because things happened in my favor that wouldn't have happened if I wasn't a doctor.

A lab guy came in at 2:00 in the morning to check my hemoglobin while I had two units of blood hanging — one in each arm.

I said, "I don't think you want to check my hemoglobin right now because I'm getting blood."

"It's ordered for 2:00," he said.

"This is not the time to do it. It's not going to be accurate. Check with the nurse."

"But I really need to do it now."

I was almost too sick to get angry, but not quite, and I had had enough of that thoughtless rule following. I said, "Then why don't you just draw it out of the blood bag? You'll get the same damn reading."

He ran off and, I guess, asked the nurse, because he didn't come back.

Another night a tech came in wanting to dose me with some medicine and couldn't figure out how fast to run the IV. She was supposed to give me eighty milligrams of medicine over ten hours, and she couldn't get eighty milligrams programmed into the machine.

"Why," I said, "don't you punch in eight milligrams per hour for ten hours?"

"That sounds right, I guess. Are you sure? I just can't figure it out."

"Just attach the pump and set it for eight milligrams an hour. It'll be fine."

I don't know how that would have worked out if I wasn't a doctor.

And about the fifth day they were trying to figure out why I was still bleeding so they were going to do an endoscopy and put a camera down my throat. They took me downstairs.

The nurse said, "Have you ever had a colonoscopy?"

I said, "Yes, I have, but I'm not having one today."

She said, "Oh, yes, you are."

I said, "Nooo, I'm not. I'm having an endoscopy."

She looked at my chart then looked me over and said, "I'm pretty sure you're having a colonoscopy."

"Call upstairs."

She reluctantly called, nodded a few times, then put down the phone and turned the bed around. It was another time that I was glad I was a doctor. What did patients do who had no pull? What did they do when they couldn't understand the technicalities of what they were being told? I was seeing my world from the patient's point of view in a way I never had before — a deeper, emotional way. I had known the way patients' fears sounded; now I knew how they felt.

I had always been skeptical about medical authority, maybe because I was so old when I entered that world. And you see things over the years that make you value your own instincts over what someone else tells you. In my workaholic days a few years before the knee surgery, I went through a bout of atrial fibrillation. There are a lot of ways that the heart can beat erratically, and they call for different therapies. So the cardiologist had me wear a halter monitor — a small electronic recorder that sends a record of the heartbeat to a monitoring center. When I had an episode of my heart misfiring I'd press a little button and in a few minutes I'd get a call from somewhere in Kansas.

The guy from Kansas said, "What were you doing when it happened?"

"Reading a book."

"How did you feel when it happened?"

"Kind of lightheaded."

"Okay, reset your monitor."

And that would be it. The same routine, over and over every day for a couple of weeks. I began to wonder if it made any difference what I said. So the next time I missed a few beats and the guy asked me what I had been doing I said, "I was sound asleep and when I woke up it felt like an elephant was sitting on my chest. I had terrible pain shooting down my left arm and my heart was going a mile a minute. I'm covered in sweat."

"Okay, reset your monitor."

I finally called my cardiologist and told him that he needed to talk to his monitoring people. We got it straightened out, but it confirmed that strain of doubt I have about blindly doing what you're told to do without questioning it.

So when I finally got the people at the hospital to put the camera in the right end, the endoscopy revealed two ulcers. One was old — probably from right after the knee surgery and one was still oozing. They decided not to cauterize (sear and seal) the new ulcer because it wasn't bleeding much and cauterizing can — rarely — cause problems. It was a perfect case of hiding from possible litigation. The surgeons had been right there. All they needed to do was seal the ulcer.

I got six more units of blood after that. That's a lot of blood. I had received two units of blood a day for seven straight days. It was my entire blood volume. After six units my hemoglobin was 4. By Sunday night I was in bad shape. It was the longest night of my life. Nothing they tried had worked, and I decided that I was going to die. I just couldn't see how this was ever going to end. They kept giving me blood and my hemoglobin kept dropping. Through some stroke of luck, though, that night I got a nurse who, I'm sure, saved my life.

Sunday night around 10:00 they tried to give me my ninth unit of blood and had to call in the IV team because they were out of veins. I had had enough. There seemed to be no way out of this cycle of IVs, bleeding, and more IVs. There's a dangerous psychological place that patients can go to when hopelessness takes over. I've seen it before in patients and the results aren't good. Then a nurse I'd never seen before came on duty, and there was something about her that reassured me. She was crisp and decisive in her movements, smart and incisive with her questions.

She worked with the IV team to help them find a vein and then hung the blood. There was trouble getting the blood started, and she was in there every ten minutes adjusting the blood bags. She was supremely competent, confident, and upbeat. She made me feel better just being around her, though at that point I was so down that apparently any improvement didn't show.

She asked, "What's wrong with you, Doctor? Why are you so depressed?"

"I decided tonight that this isn't going to work. The bleeding just isn't going to stop. I'm not going to make it."

She shook her head and said, "Look, I know you're frustrated and tired. But you're not dying on my watch, I won't allow it. So there's no more of that talk. Okay?"

"Okay," I agreed. It was silly in a way. I've seen enough death in hospitals. It can come quickly despite good practice. But her matter-of-fact strength and humanity touched me and did give me strength. She was in and out of that room constantly all night, checking my readings, checking the blood bags, giving them strategic pokes. With every visit she included a little pep talk. I drifted in and out of sleep and as dawn approached I was feeling better. Singlehandedly she had pulled me out of that dangerous mental place.

I will forever be indebted to that superb nurse, Chelsea Greene. I'm in debt, too, to that entire horrible experience. Because of it, I believe that I became a better doctor than all the seminars, courses, and medical experience I had had before that had made me. I had been in search of the ability to see for a long time. But I hadn't understood what that meant in its fullest sense. I had thought of "what was in front of me" as a medical condition, a set of circumstances and symptoms, a story. It is all that. What I had not appreciated fully was Vic Fortin's deep wisdom: you're not treating a medical problem, you're treating a person with a medical problem. Oh, I thought I knew that. Like a lot of things we know, though, I knew only the words, not the emotional truth. Now I knew a little of what it meant to be helpless and not taken seriously — weak in every sense. Scared, very nearly, to death.

I say I knew "a little" because, whatever I experienced, I was still a doctor! I thought of what it truly meant to be a clinic patient — sick, scared, and powerless, lying in a dark room late at night with a heart full of fear. There's no way, simply through training and best practices to deal with the deep anguish a patient feels. Professional competence has to be combined with simple human sympathy. Vic Fortin knew that; Chelsea Greene knew that. Two of my teachers.

Chapter 17

Death and Dying

In Which I Learn to Deal with Loss

My brush with dying taught me that my own death and the deaths of others are two quite different things. At a couple of points during my crisis, death seemed an acceptable option. Maybe that's the body's way of preparing the mind for the inevitable. Luckily for me, the inevitable was sent packing — first by a bunch of firefighters and EMTs and later by a feisty nurse.

The deaths of others are harder to handle. So many human beings seem to be wired to save others. When our strange species isn't doing terrible things to each other, we're trying to save each other. It's there in the news stories about rescues and self-sacrifice. One of the prime motives that drives people into the medical world is that urge to help, and, if possible, heal.

Watching others die is one of the least bearable of human experiences and when those others have given you their trust and are under your care their loss is excruciating. If the caregivers allow those losses to take too much of a toll, though, the caregivers' effectiveness is weakened.

I lost my first patient a half hour into my med school clinicals. It was the first time I was in a hospital as something other than a patient. I had just moved from the second-year classroom onto the hospital floor, and I was working with a one-armed intern. Kathy had lost her left arm in an accident and had a noticeable chip on the remaining shoulder. She was a tough customer, but I could understand why. There weren't that many two-armed female interns in those days. Women were discouraged and disparaged by the medical establishment and a disability could only make it worse. Kathy made it to where she was because she was very good; she knew she had to be.

Fifteen minutes into our first rounds together we got a code blue from radiology and we had no idea how to get there. We got directions from a nurse, started running down the stairs, and when we got to the radiology floor the door was locked. We ran down one more flight, followed a hallway, went back up a floor and found the unit. There was a seventeen-year-old girl there with stage four breast cancer who had been getting chemo when she went into respiratory arrest. Soon there were six of us — the fourth-year sub-intern and three more of my fellow third-years. We started CPR — Kathy pushed on her chest and I did the breathing until the anesthesiologist got there and intubated her. It made no difference. Her lungs were shot. She died while we watched.

We were all hit hard and after the frenzy of orders and procedures, we just stood there in silence. My head was spinning from the CPR and stress. (Interestingly, today we tell doctors that one of the first things to do during a code is to take your own pulse. Overexcitement is dangerous to the patient and can cause bad decisions and rough, clumsy movements.) I had watched helplessly as her vitals on the monitors dropped and disappeared, and over thirty years later I remember exactly how it felt — a mixture of horror, impotence, sadness, anger, and guilt. There is often, as with that young woman, nothing that can be done to avoid death. But that's logical, and your deepest reaction is always emotional.

After she died, I sleepwalked out of the room and nearly collided with her brother. Kathy was still in the room finishing up the code, and it was left to me to tell him. He didn't look much older than his sister, and I thought he was going to hit me. He had been crying, and he punched the wall near my head and put a hole in the plaster. I wanted to tell him that I was frustrated and angry, too, but it was hard to find the right words. It still is.

There are different kinds of deaths; some are expected and some sudden, some unbearable, and some merciful. Most doctors never get used to the emotional consequences, but they do get better at handling them. You learn how to compartmentalize — how to keep your attention on the task at hand whether it's finishing a procedure, speaking to family members, filling out forms, or just getting down the hall to where you need to be next. Focus on the tasks at hand, and you can minimize thinking about the loss. For the new doctor who hasn't developed their go-to coping skills, it's hard. I try to teach young residents that it's the patient who had the disease. We didn't cause it, and we did our best to cure it. That rationalization only goes so far, though. I've had many residents cry on my shoulder quite literally. I feel like crying sometimes, but I think the old-timers need to hold it together for the sake of those around us. The drive home is another matter.

OBs have it better than a lot of doctors because our patients tend to be healthy young women and the mortality rate is low. But precisely because the patients are young and healthy losing them seems worse. Losing a baby is devastating. In obstetrics, most infant deaths happen before birth and are caused by prematurity or birth defects. They're stillborn. Every year we get better outcomes because technology and training are getting better, but during my days of med school and residency, we didn't have a lot of prenatal diagnostic tools. Ultrasound was new and, unless you were a Vic Fortin, it was difficult to make a diagnosis with it. We did amniocenteses but got less information from them. Now we can collect genetic material, take a couple of weeks to grow genes, and construct a baby's entire genome — a full set of forty-six chromosomes. You can look at them on something like a piece of film. In the old days, we did a chemical analysis of the amniotic fluid to look for lung maturity or signs of a threatening miscarriage. The hormone estriol was a cue of possible problems as was

Alpha-Fetoprotein. AFP told us if the baby had a neural tube defect and was leaking cerebral or spinal fluid. If the reading was high that was suspicious. And we only looked at highs; low readings were thought to be irrelevant.

An interesting story is the way a relationship between a low AFP and Down syndrome was discovered. One day in the 1980s in a Cleveland pediatrician's office two women were talking and they both had a child with Down's. They started comparing experiences and at some point one of the mothers said, "You know, I had a low AFP and I've always wondered if that had something to do with my baby having Down's."

The other woman said, "Yes! I had a low AFP, and they told me it was nothing to worry about."

They told the pediatrician, and he decided to look into it. Eventually a study was done, and it turned out that about a third of the babies with Down's have low AFPs. So we look at the low readings, too.

I diagnosed cancer in a baby at twenty-eight weeks when I was doing an ultrasound. That's rare, thank God. The mother saw me measuring the growth and asked what we were looking at. I had to tell her that her baby had a big tumor. Then she asked me if it was malignant, and I said that with a growth that size at that baby's age it probably was. She was horrified, but I couldn't lie. We were going to wait until she was term and deliver the baby, then see if there was anything we could do. It died a few weeks later, though.

A similar thing happened when a patient and I watched her fetus die on the ultrasound monitor. She tensed and asked me, "Did the heart just stop?"

I said, "Yes, I'm waiting for it to start up again." It didn't. The baby was too young to do any kind of emergency C-section. That was truly awful.

That also raises a difficult question about emergency procedures and medical ethics. When a C-section is done, the doctor gives the mother all sorts of morbidity. There's danger there so you'd better be damned sure that it's worth it. Those are some of the toughest decisions we make. What if a woman comes in and she's bleeding? An ultrasound shows that the heartbeat isn't there or is very slow. What do you do? Is it too late or not? I remember seeing an attending that I thought was brave. He got called into the delivery room on an emergency, and they told him that there was no heartbeat on the baby. They were getting ready to do a stat section.

"Hold your horses," he said. "We're not doing a C-section for a dead baby." That takes a lot of guts.

A doctor increases the risk for the mother with a C-section, but things are a lot better than they used to be. Maternal deaths are rare these days, about three in ten thousand, and the causes tend to be catastrophic — pulmonary embolisms or hemorrhage. Those are the unexpected deaths. I remember one young mother who died while I was on vacation. I came back to the news and all I could think about was the smile she had on her face the last time I saw her.

Another tough case happened while I was off duty. I came on call at 7:00 a.m. and a young Somali woman had died about an hour earlier from a massive brain injury. She was post-partum and had been complaining about a headache. When she went into seizures everyone thought it was eclampsia, but she had herniated her brain stem and there was nothing to be done. It was so odd for a person her age that we thought she must have had a brain tumor. The postmortem revealed an anatomical defect that was congenital.

The Somali community is close. Her room and the hallway outside were filled with family members and friends. They were terribly upset, of course, and I think some of them blamed the doctors. But there was an older relative who took me aside and told me that her mother had died the same way. A day after this patient had been born, her mother fell ill and died in the hospital of a brain herniation. And the baby that we had delivered the day before was a girl.

I talked to the husband through an interpreter and tried to explain that his daughter might have the same condition. There wasn't much trust there, however. I don't know if he thought that we were trying to make excuses for the death, but I'm afraid that that little girl may never understand the pattern of her mother's and grandmother's deaths and how she fits into it. She probably should not have children. It would be hard to convince a religious

Somalian of that, though. They would probably want to rely on Allah's will.

One of the major shortcomings of medical education, I think, is that no one teaches doctors how to handle death or failure. Many doctors don't know how to deal with patients they can't help — either in terms of counseling them or in counseling themselves. When a patient comes to you with something you can't fix you're never told that you can't do anything about that. Doctors are trained to always look for something to do, some curative strategy. Even when oncologists know they're beaten I've seen them put their patient through another round of tests or some stopgap operation. We simply don't accept death in American medicine. When people come to us with a horrible problem that we can't fix we still try. That kind of rote persistence can come close to violating our oath to do no harm.

A personal consequence of close familiarity with death is that a doctor often becomes the go-to person in his or her family when death intrudes. When my father was dying of a neurological disease, we found out that he had about two years to live. I was the one who had to tell everyone. The assumption is, I guess, that a doctor can answer questions more authoritatively and won't be disturbed by the presence of death in the family. I guess I'm authoritative, but the death affects me the same as anyone else. Though I don't resent having to be the intermediary for the rest of the family I think others could do the job, too. Dad's death was hard for me, but at least it was a quiet and long-expected death. My sister's was the hardest; she was murdered.

Mary Pat and I were "Irish twins." I was born in January, and Mary Pat was born the following December. So we were always close. We called each other often. Sometimes she rang me as I was reaching for the phone to punch in her number. One Sunday night I came home from the hospital and my niece, Katrina, called. "I can't find Mom. She's usually home on Sunday night and I'm really getting worried."

Katrina had been calling friends and driving around likely places for five hours, so I got worried, too. I went to the Worthington police near Mary Pat's home, and they told me that there was nothing they could do. Five hours seemed as short to them as it felt long to us. I also told them that my niece had found her mother's car at her boyfriend's place in West Jefferson, on the other side of town and there was no answer at the door or on the phone.

"We can't do anything about West Jefferson," said the cop. "You'll have to go out there to the police."

"Can't you at least call them and tell them about the car being found and that we're afraid?"

"No, we can't do that. Tell them yourself."

I was angry as I ran to the car and drove the twenty miles to West Jefferson. I called my son Patrick on the way and asked him to come with me. I didn't know what I was going to do. Maybe I had visions of storming the apartment to rescue my sister. I also called Tony, my lawyer brother.

Tony said, "Don't tell me anything you're going to do because I can't have prior knowledge of it."

That scared me a little and slowed me down a lot. The tough guy approach wasn't necessary, though, because when Patrick and I got there the police had taken my niece to the station and asked us to wait there while they checked out the apartment. It was a relief that they were taking us seriously, but it was a terrible ninety-minute wait. When they got back, the officers told us that Mary Pat and the boyfriend were both dead. He strangled her then shot himself — apparently the deaths happened twenty-four hours apart. What was he thinking about for twenty-four hours?

I beat myself up for months trying to decide if I could have prevented the murder. There were signs of problems, but they weren't the kind I was able to read at that point. They had dated for seven years; he had never had a history of violence. I never heard him raise his voice to my sister. He killed my sister when she was a week shy of her fifty-seventh birthday.

I wish I could say that Mary Pat's death gave me a deeper understanding of death. It didn't, but what it did do was give me a clearer eye to see domestic abuse and adamant motivation to combat it. Doctors deal with domestic violence all the time. We're taught to look for it because a high percentage of women who come into the ER are victims. They don't tell you that they are. They tell you that they fell down the steps or slipped on ice or had some other kind of accident. The doctor often has to dig for the truth, and sometimes the truth doesn't appear until it's too late to help.

After the murder, I became far better in practical ways at handling domestic violence cases. Recognizing the physical symptoms of abuse is only the start for a physician. It's just as important to become familiar with the psychological symptoms and the patterns of behavior that characterize both the victim and the abuser.

I know now that possessiveness is a strong predictor of violence. The abuser may never have harmed his victim physically, but if he has been jealous and controlling the triggers are set for something dangerous to happen. Mary Pat's boyfriend was unusually possessive. He was fixated on where she was and who she was seeing. On days when they were apart, he called her twice an hour. His constant phone calls and relentless suspicion finally became unbearable and my sister ended the relationship, but he asked her to wait until after the holidays. This is textbook behavior for potential violence. Delaying a breakup is dangerous for the abused. He was strangely pleasant to me at Thanksgiving dinner — another red flag that no one saw. I was puzzled. Now I think he had decided at that point what he was going to do; the extra time allowed him to plan it. His friendliness at Thanksgiving was the eerie calm before the storm. The possessive person will never accept the idea that what he sees as his possession will belong to someone else. Violence or death comes next.

I had a patient right after Mary Pat died who came in because of pre-term labor. She was at risk for delivery, but she was also at risk from her boyfriend at home. He was beating her. So we admitted her for the pre-term labor, but really as a way to protect her from the abuser. I talked to her and tried to use my family's experience to sway her. It didn't work. She wouldn't even ban him from her hospital room; they had vocal arguments even there.

She had her baby and was home about a month when the boyfriend called the police and told them that he had killed her and the body was in the kitchen. That's the awful thing I learned from the death of Mary Pat. It's so very hard to protect the abused from the abuser. Love, fear, intimidation, and need come together in a tragic way.

After Mary Pat's death, I was the one who took my niece home, told her in-laws, and called the rest of the family and closest friends. Years later I ran into a distant relative who identified me as the one who always calls with the bad news.

That's okay. I accept the role. I am far more used to death than anyone else in the family, and I want to keep it that way. It is a weight, though, just as it is at the hospital.

My mother-in-law took a little of the shine off my reputation as an expert. When she was dying Nancy and her sisters kept asking me when she was going to go. I would give them a guess, and Helen keep hanging on. I finally stopped predicting her death and one night I told Nancy's sister Beth that she could go home and get a shower. I was sitting there in Helen's room reading the paper when I looked over and she was gone. Wrong again. Helen would have chuckled about that.

Enough about death. Dwelling on it is like staring at the sun; too long a look can blind you. It's the ultimate failure for a doctor. As heavy as the burden of death can be for us, though, we have a wonderful counterweight. We save lives, too. OBs have it the best when they can rescue a baby. I tell internists that they only save the last few years of a patient's life. We save the whole damn thing.

Making a difference in people's lives was why I went into medicine and looking back over the years as I wrote this book allowed me to see myself coming closer and closer to becoming the doctor I wanted to be. I may not have the balletic skills with a scalpel that John Gibbons had or the psychic diagnostic ability of Vic Fortin, but I'm learning. When making a difference means saving a life, it's the best.

Chapter 18

That Guy

In Which I Finally Learn to See What's in Front of Me

I wanted to be that guy. Ever since the night Nancy and I saw *Coming Home* I wanted to be that guy — the one who gets called in on the tough problems. The doctor who's seen it all and knows what to do. The one who sees what's there and not what's expected or feared. I hope that doesn't sound like conceit. Or male ego. I've worked with great women, both doctors and nurses, who wanted that same thing and got it. It's that drive to do something of worth, to make a difference in people's lives, and to do it with confidence and grace. Becoming that person, though, is such a slow process that the recognition of it can be surprising.

When I had been at St. Ann's for five years or so, I was walking down a hall on our Ob-Gyn floor, and as I went by an open door I heard a heartbeat that wasn't as fast as it should have been. At this point in my career I'm able to hear a monitor from the hall and recognize the heart rate, and this one was too slow. A baby's rate is supposed to be from 120 to 160 beats per minute.

When it's 90 like this one was, something's wrong — or they're listening to the mom. I looked inside the room and one of our family practice residents was trying to put a fetal scalp electrode on the baby. It's an electronic contact hooked to a little screw that's attached to the baby's scalp. He was having a terrible time and said,

"Dr. Kington, I can't get this electrode to stay on. It keeps getting washed out."

It was a classic case of seeing the trees and not the forest. The heartbeat was 90 and the fluid that was washing out the electrode was blood. I said,

"Zack, she's hemorrhaging. We need to do a section right now!"

The mom had what's called a vasa previa — the blood vessels go to the placenta over the birth membranes, and when the water breaks the vessels rupture. The baby was bleeding out, not the mom. Babies don't have that much blood, so we didn't have that much time.

We rushed the mom into the OR and sectioned her, but the baby had lost so much blood she was almost transparent. The NICU people resuscitated her for eighteen minutes. I was sure that little girl was gone, but they got her reversed and she ended up fine. Those are the kinds of things that get you over the bad places. When I was a resident there was no way that I could have recognized from the hall what that heart rate meant. And I could easily have gotten so intent on the importance of that scalp electrode that I missed the life-threatening symptoms literally washing over me. At some point that resident will be where he needs to be — where all the good doctors I learned from were. That's what experience can do if you let it.

Being the guy who gets called can be great for the self-esteem, but bad for the nerves. I was finally the oldest, most experienced doctor in the hospital, but who could I turn to when I got stuck? It can get lonely. I got a call at home one afternoon from our chief resident, Helen McCann. She asked me if I had ever seen a case of necrotizing fasciitis, the so-called "flesh-eating bacteria." I told her that I had seen some cases before and gave her advice, but I could tell from the way she was answering that she wanted me there, so I put away the lawn mower and came in. On the way over my emotions were bouncing between the great feeling of being relied upon and the fear of facing a dangerous situation.

I could see right away that it was "nec fasc." The infection has the striking presentation of dead necrotized tissue surrounding a gaping wound. The bacteria destroy fat, muscle tissue, and the fascia or tough layer that surrounds the muscles. The nerves are necrotized as well, and the result is one of the hallmarks of the infection. The patient can't feel the wound. Usually when someone has an infection and cellulitis it's extremely painful. Not with nec fasc.

I learned much of what I know about necrotizing fasciitis from a patient — the lack of sensation in particular. It had been about five years before this case, and like Helen's patient, the infection had invaded her C-section incision. She was a fearless and articulate woman who was able to tell me useful detail about her symptoms and sensations. The other primary sign of nec fasc is a crackling noise when the tissues are pressed. Such "crepitance" is caused by tiny bubbles of gas that formed in the dead tissue by the anaerobic bacteria causing the disease. Most commonly, the bacteria are a type of strep called Group A, but there are other strains that can necrotize tissue. Clostridium is another. These are not exotic bacteria. We interact with them all the time and generally the problems they cause aren't dangerous. Strep throat, for example, can be painful and annoying, but if treated isn't usually life-threatening. What causes an infection to make that fatal jump? The condition of one's immune system and genetics play a role. My first case of a necrotizing infection was the result of genetic disposition.

When I was a new attending at Ohio State, we had a patient who gave birth then got an infection in her episiotomy incision that began killing her tissues. The lab identified the pathogen as a clostridium strain, but we didn't have any experience with it. Nobody seemed to. There were only four cases reported in the literature, and they were described in one paper by a Korean doctor. We called him overseas and told him that we had a patient with that unusual clostridium infection.

He asked, "Is she Asian?"

"Yes," we said.

"Well, then, she's going to die."

We were shocked and annoyed by what seemed callous self-assurance and told him that she wasn't in such bad shape at the moment. She was in the ICU and appeared to be responding to antibiotics.

"Yes," he said. "That sounds consistent. But tomorrow she'll probably get worse, then go into a coma, and in forty-eight hours she'll be dead. We've never been able to treat this."

And that's what happened. Apparently there's a small group of Asian people with a genetic disposition that makes them susceptible to this infection. Their bodies can't fight it off. So my first experience with a necrotizing fasciitis was sad and frustrating. The best we could do was tell the family her prognosis and give them the opportunity to say goodbye. Helen's patient fared better. The antibiotics finally stopped the spread of the infection, and we left the wound open until the plastic surgeons could go in later and fix it.

The times I've been called in as last resort have seldom been dangerous or tragic, I'm glad to say. Most of the cases involved my skill with older delivery techniques that are being lost. Fundal pressure is one such technique — pressing down on the fundus, or top part of the uterus, to help deliver a baby vaginally. In a nine-month pregnant woman that would be right up under the rib cage. It helps the mother deliver a more powerful push. When she's pushing and not getting there you can reach a critical point. Maybe the baby's heart rate goes down or it's in danger of being infected. Sometimes you just have to get the baby out, and the choices are delivering vaginally or doing a C-section. The question is always, "Which way is going to be faster?" As I've mentioned, C-sections can open up dangerous consequences and need to remain the doctor's Plan B.

Fundal pressure can cause problems, though, and is a controversial technique. Most problems happened to the nurses doing the fundal pressure technique. The nurses came away with rotator cuff injuries, shoulder problems, and sprained wrists. You have to push pretty hard. I've seen people doing fundal pressure with an elbow or a knee which can present problems for the patient. It's difficult to control pressure that way. There are great big veins that run across the sides of the uterus that can hemorrhage if they're damaged. It's also possible to puncture the uterine wall. That's why it's better to use the hands, and that's where my size helps. I can't count how many times during an initial interview that the patient has recognized my fundal pressure technique.

"I remember you, Doc. You helped deliver my last baby. You climbed up on my belly and pushed."

Most of those who taught me how to do fundal pressure were nurses. Now they're generally not allowed to do it. No hospital wants a nurse on worker's comp. Once I learned it, I relied on it and now I get relied upon by others. That feels good. A resident, Justin Hindman, named me "The Fundal Bear" at some point in my career and the name stuck. It's good to get called in to a problem delivery and to be able to give the final word on whether a kid can be delivered vaginally. "No, this one's too big." "This one might need forceps." "This one might need some gentle fundal." When I was a resident at St. Francis, we would talk to Tony Vintzileos about problem deliveries and what we should do. He would say, "GTBO." Get the baby out. That's one of the things I've learned how to do.

When you're the one who gets called, though, there can be some awkward social situations. Usually it's the doctor who's calling and that makes it easy. You're simply coming in to help. John Gibbons used to say that when you're called in to assist the first thing you say to the doctor is, "Well, it looks pretty bad, but I'll see what I can do."

Then if you don't succeed it's expected and if you do you're a hero. That was maybe the only suggestion of Gibbons's that I never used. I thought it made people feel bad.

Sometimes the nurse called for help for someone else and that's always a dicey political situation. Some attendings have too much pride, and they resent the call for help. It's a trait that you don't want in a doctor, and it's something that we try to address in training residents. One of the best things you can do when you get in trouble is call for help. You can be so close to the problem that you buy into one view of the situation and can't think straight. A bit of terror makes the situation even worse.

Being the bearer of lost techniques is a peculiar role. A lot of the older ways of doing medicine don't deserve to survive.

They've died for a reason, and I'm happy that they're gone. But fundal pressure, along with the careful use of forceps to help with problem deliveries, shouldn't have been lost. It happened because of the litigious society we live in and the bottom-line approach of modern hospitals. Fundal pressure and forceps use require a lot of training and experience. Best practice training these days is as quick and efficient as it can be. Learning nuances isn't cost effective, and there's that lawsuit lurking if there are problems. The result is unneeded C-sections and an open door to real problems.

So I'm The Fundal Bear. I've become the guy. It feels great, but it's temporary. Someone else will take my place with a different background and skill set. The experience will be there, though, and that hard-won capacity to see what's in front of you. And not all the tradition bearers will be doctors. Our great nurse Amy is skilled with fundal pressure and has used it effectively in a lot of tricky cases. Those gifted caregivers, doctors and nurses both, are out there. It was Amy who gave me the most valuable medical award I've ever received. We were rushing to yet another tough delivery when she turned to me and said, "Promise me that you'll never retire."

That kind of acknowledgement from a colleague and a seasoned pro isn't as flashy as a plaque or a certificate or an engraved watch, but it's more meaningful than all those things together.

Epilogue

I had just opened the door to my office on a Monday morning when I got a call from Beth Rogers, one of our third-year residents, about a problem delivery. Beth had been a pleasure to teach and was one of my favorites. She was bright, she listened, and she knew how to take what she had learned and adapt it to different situations. Now she just sounded tired and worried.

"Dr. Kington, I need your help with this case. I just got in here and we have a patient who we've been trying to induce all weekend. I think it's a tubal pregnancy. Can you come up and take a look?"

A tubal pregnancy is an ectopic pregnancy in which the fetus develops outside the uterus — in this case the fallopian tube. At some point the growth of the fetus ruptures the tube and there's hemorrhaging. If Beth was right her patient could be in danger.

Beth showed me the ultrasounds and said, "It's a miscarriage, but look at the size of that fetus. It measures around fourteen weeks. That's way too big to be a tubal. And it's too big for a D and C, so they were trying to induce labor, but it's not working."

She put down the ultrasounds and looked at me. "I think it *is* an ectopic. I remember you once told us that if you couldn't induce labor you should consider that the baby might not be in the uterus."

I remembered that exchange. It wasn't hard. That's one of my standard-issue pearls of wisdom. I'm usually talking about a full-term pregnancy, though. Beth had something else. Fourteen weeks put that pregnancy just out of the first trimester and tubals rarely go beyond eight or nine weeks. At that point the tube ruptures. So what was this? Beth had the likeliest answer.

As many times as I've mentioned ectopic pregnancies, I'm not sure I've gotten across how tough they are to deal with. Sometimes I feel like I spent half my career trying to figure out if an ER patient had one. It's not as simple as it seems. You see a woman in her first trimester, and she has pain or bleeding or both. You look for the pregnancy and you can't find it, then you look at the blood work to see what the numbers are doing. Those are the levels of human chorionic gonadotropin — more specifically, the beta subunit of that protein. Beta HCG is the protein that's looked for in pregnancy tests. If it's up, you're pregnant; if it's zero, you're not pregnant.

With ectopics we have to look at the trend because the levels themselves are unreliable. They rise for a while until about ten weeks then they drop off. Beta HGC is supposed to be doubling in a normal pregnancy, while in an ectopic pregnancy the numbers could double, or stay the same, or drop, or do anything. It's easy to rule *in* a normal pregnancy after a couple of doublings because you see the pattern and eventually you see the fetus. But if you don't have those doublings it's hard to figure out where the baby is. Is the patient miscarrying? Is it a tubal pregnancy? While the doctor is trying to figure out the situation the patient could hemorrhage or worse.

"Let's take a look," I said, and when we did another ultrasound I could tell that the fetus was not in the uterus. Looking closely, I could see the uterine wall. This fetus wasn't behind it. Beth was right. It was lying on top of the uterus — a tubal pregnancy, and the biggest one I had ever seen. It was in the end of the tube, where the fimbria (the fringes of tissue around the fallopian tubes) are like a flower. This fetus had succumbed because the tissues around it weren't supplying enough nutrients for a fetus that large. So while I watched, Beth did a laparoscopy, removed the fetus, and fixed the tube. Her surgical technique was sure and confident, but what impressed me more was the way she had moved beyond the ambiguous ultrasounds and wrong diagnosis of the weekend residents to recognize the ectopic pregnancy. I'm glad I was there to listen to her ideas and second the diagnosis, but if I hadn't been there she would have done the right thing. She had taken a practical tip that I had told her, used it in a different context, and saw a problem that others had missed.

As it did with me, though, that ability to see came slowly. I remember a very different Beth just two years earlier when she was doing one of her first C-sections. Like a lot of inexperienced operators, Beth had been too energetic in her use of the scalpel and had sliced into the patient's bladder. There, bobbing around in clear sight, was the balloon tip of a Foley catheter, which was draining urine. Beth had seen a Foley hundreds of times in her training, but she stared at this one without a flicker of recognition.

"What in the world?" she said. "What *is* that?"

"What's it look like?"

"I don't know! I mean, it looks like a Foley, but it couldn't be."

"Why not?"

"Because the Foley is in the bladder!"

"Right."

I couldn't see much of Beth's face above the surgical mask, but I saw her eyes close for a second in embarrassment. Then she called for some suture to repair her mistake. Beth was a self-possessed and dignified young doctor even then (John Gibbons would have loved her). I didn't like putting her on the spot with my Socratic questioning, but I wanted her to see the Foley herself. That little snap in which the world rushed into focus was worth a lot more than me telling her what I saw.

Now Beth had become a good doctor. That had been a smart and sensitive bit of diagnosis. It might have saved a life. If they had sat and waited for further developments on that patient one of the developments could have been a major hemorrhage. As I walked back down to my office I thought of Big Ed Fields and the way he ignored lab reports when his instincts told him the truth. I thought of Vic Fortin and how he could read the murkiest of ultrasounds and nail the exact diagnosis. I think more these days of the great doctors who taught me, and the older I get the more I appreciate how much I'm a part of the long chain of medical knowledge. Generations of doctors speak to today's physicians through those my age. Those young doctors, in turn, will speak to those who follow.

It doesn't matter how much techniques and technology have transformed medicine; the necessity of seeing is still at the center of the art. Whatever procedure doctors are using, whatever new tool they're employing, the importance of the practical insight is still there. Doctors are relentlessly schooled, and, yes, the brain must guide the hands. But each case has something to teach, something to interpret and understand, that can't be learned from a book. The simple ability to see what's in front of you — Beth had it now and one day she would pass on her ability to see to another young doctor. I hope in another thirty years watching that gift play out before her would make her as proud of her resident as I was of her.

The End

Acknowledgments

Over the years Kevin would tell me his great stories and always end by saying, "That's one for the Kington Chronicles." Finally I said, "Let's write that damn book." So we did, and it took more time and work than either of us expected. Something else I didn't expect was the gift of getting to know Kevin and Nancy better through the process of revisiting their lives, and I think even more of them now than before we started writing. Perhaps that's one definition of a well-lived life. And I find that no matter how many times I reread the stories I still enjoy them. That's all Kevin. I thank him for that, and the opportunity he gave me to write the chronicles with him.

I want to thank those who read the manuscript in progress as they were crucial in making it a better book: Toni and Fred Johnson, and Sonia Kovitz. I also want to thank Peter who edited our photographs at the eleventh hour. I especially want to thank our writing coach and editor, Susan Simmons. Her great ear and clear eye have made this book better in every sense. Her patience isn't bad, either. Huge thanks to all. Whatever problems with accuracy or quality that remain in this book are in spite of their help. ~ Jas

CR

About the Authors ...

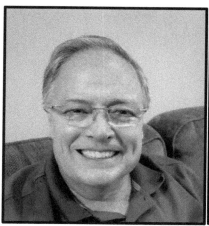 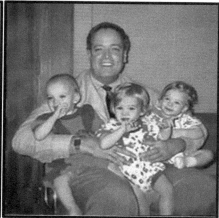

Kevin Kington, M.D., is a retired obstetrician/gynecologist who lives with his wife Nancy in Columbus, Ohio. He attended medical school at The Ohio State University and enjoyed a 30-year career as a doctor and teacher. When not telling stories, he golfs, plays bridge, chauffeurs grandchildren, and practices the guitar.

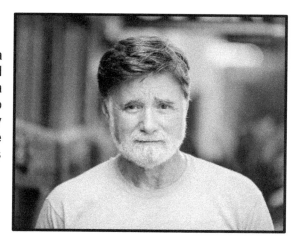

Jas Scarff is a writer, folklorist, and musician. He is a graduate of Ohio Wesleyan University and The Ohio State University and lives in Columbus, Ohio.

CPSIA information can be obtained
at www.ICGtesting.com
Printed in the USA
LVHW080253081118
596404LV00017B/501/P